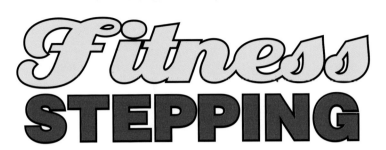

STEPPING

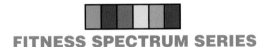

FITNESS SPECTRUM SERIES

Debi Pillarella
Scott O. Roberts

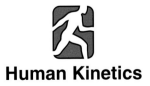

Human Kinetics

ᵒging-in-Publication Data

t O. Roberts.
      p.   cm. -- (Fitness spectrum series)
   Includes index.
   ISBN 0-87322-835-9
   1. Step aerobics.   I. Roberts, Scott.   II. Title.   III. Series.
   GV501.5.B35   1996
   613.7'1--dc20   96-1625
                                                          CIP

ISBN: 0-87322-835-9

Copyright © 1996 by Human Kinetics Publishers, Inc.

Developmental Editor: Kirby Mittelmeier; **Assistant Editor:** Chad Johnson; **Editorial Assistant:** Amy Carnes; **Copyeditor:** Holly Gilly; **Proofreader:** Erin Cler; **Indexer:** Theresa Schaefer; **Typesetter and Layout Artist:** Francine Hamerski; **Text Designer:** Keith Blomberg; **Photo Editor:** Boyd LaFoon; **Cover Designer:** Jack Davis; **Photographer (cover):** Tom McCarthy/Unicorn; **Photographer (interior):** Chris Brown; **Illustrator:** Studio 2-D

Human Kinetics books are available at special discounts for bulk purchase. Special editions or book excerpts can also be created to specification. For details, contact the Special Sales Manager at Human Kinetics.

Printed in Hong Kong   10   9   8   7   6   5   4   3   2   1

Human Kinetics
Web site: http://www.humankinetics.com/

United States: Human Kinetics, P.O. Box 5076, Champaign, IL 61825-5076
1-800-747-4457
e-mail: humank@hkusa.com

Canada: Human Kinetics, Box 24040, Windsor, ON N8Y 4Y9
1-800-465-7301 (in Canada only)
e-mail: humank@hkcanada.com

Europe: Human Kinetics, P.O. Box IW14, Leeds LS16 6TR, United Kingdom
(44) 1132 781708
e-mail: humank@hkeurope.com

Australia: Human Kinetics, 57A Price Avenue, Lower Mitcham, South Australia 5062
(08) 277 1555
e-mail: humank@hkaustralia.com

New Zealand: Human Kinetics, P.O. Box 105-231, Auckland 1
(09) 523 3462
e-mail: humank@hknewz.com

Contents

PART I

PREPARING TO STEP

Stepping up and down is part of your normal daily activities. You step using stairs, stools, ladders, and curbs, yet you probably never thought about including the up-and-down rhythm into a structured fitness program.

However, many people have discovered that stepping for fitness is not only a lot of fun and easy to do, it also has a wealth of benefits. It's lower in impact than traditional dance aerobics, burns a significant amount of calories, and doesn't require a lot of complicated choreography. As a matter of fact, stepping is one of the most popular types of aerobic exercise. We're sure that once you've gone through this book, it'll be one of your favorite types, too.

Because stepping is a natural movement, we need to focus on only a few techniques as we delve into this popular mode of training. Stepping up and down is a basic locomotor skill we learn early in life. Developing that skill into a useful type of exercise is one of the goals of this book.

The other goal is to teach you how to set up and participate in a personalized step fitness program. For example, in this book you'll find actual workouts, not just directions on technique and execution. In addition, the predesigned programs take the guesswork out of your training programs. Our workouts are diverse, flexible, and produce results. For this book to meet your personal fitness goals, we first need to look at who you are.

Maybe you're the type of person who was very fit in high school or college, but haven't worked out in years. If it's been a long time since you were highly fit, you'll need to take time and care to work into stepping shape. We'll show you how easy and enjoyable fitness stepping can be.

Perhaps you have dropped in on your neighborhood health club or YMCA for an occasional step workout, or you've joined in with your favorite exercise show celebrities and ended up feeling sore and unpleasant. We'll show you smarter and better ways to train without strain.

Maybe you're an avid stepper but you want to personalize your program to reach higher fitness goals. We'll show you how to safely challenge yourself and reach the goals you desire.

In part I, we prepare you to step right into your fitness program. We set the foundation for your future progress with this exciting program. You'll learn

- the benefits of stepping compared to other modes of training;
- how to choose proper shoes, clothing, and other equipment needed for step exercise;
- how to test your physical readiness to start a step fitness program or to adopt a more demanding training regimen;
- how to refine and perfect your stepping technique so you can move more efficiently and safely; and
- how to properly warm up, cool down, and supplement your stepping program with flexibility and strengthening exercises.

After you've learned the stepping basics, you'll delve into the color zone workouts in part II. We're sure you'll enjoy the versatility and variety of workouts in chapters 6 through 11. By following our workout schedules in part III and charting your progress, you'll be on your way to reaching your goals. We think we've said enough to whet your appetite for stepping. Read on and get ready for a fun-filled training program. Good luck!

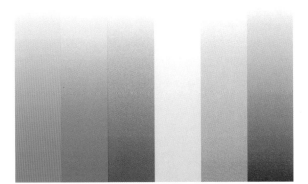

Step Aerobics for Fitness

You have walked up and down the stairs of your house, climbed a flight of stairs at the office or school, and stepped up on a curb to avoid stepping in a puddle of water countless times. You've been stepping up and down most of your life. However, it wasn't until recently that stepping as a mode of exercise hit the "big time." According to *American Fitness Magazine*, step training is the hottest fitness trend of the 1990s. Thousands of fitness enthusiasts worldwide flock to aerobic step classes weekly. The expansion of cable television and video markets has also contributed to the step aerobics boom.

Gin Miller, creative director of the Step Reebok programs, started stepping on milk crates at her home in Georgia to rehabilitate a knee injury in 1986. Since then, Gin has progressed from an avid step exerciser and step aerobics instructor to representing step aerobics worldwide. Gin has produced numerous training videos for instructors and consumers and stars on the Step Reebok cable TV show. Her expertise along with the exploding step aerobics industry have combined to be a proven winner. Gin invented an activity that is fun, effective, and adaptable to space, time, and weather constraints. Millions of others have joined her, and now you can, too.

Who Steps?

The National Sporting Goods Association reported that over 1.5 million aerobic steps were purchased in 1993 alone. In September of 1994, *Club Industry Magazine* reported nearly 7 million people participated in step aerobics.

Step aerobics shows no bias toward either sex, although more females than males participate. Approximately 16 percent of step exercisers were men and 84 percent were women, according to the National Sporting Goods Association's 1991 survey on sport participation.

Fitness stepping seems to have no age barriers either. One out of three step exercisers is between 25 and 34 years of age. Twenty-three percent are between 18 and 24 years old, and a whopping 36 percent are over age 35.

Interestingly, the National Sporting Goods Association reports that nearly one-third of the participants say they work out an average of three times a week. Such devotion to a sport must indicate it's a fun and effective way to keep fit. Richard Ban, a 65-year-old retired educator from Chicago, Illinois, his wife Josephine, who is 59 years old, and their 33-year-old daughter Michele have been enjoying step aerobics since 1988. They enjoy the simplicity, versatility, and effectiveness of the activity.

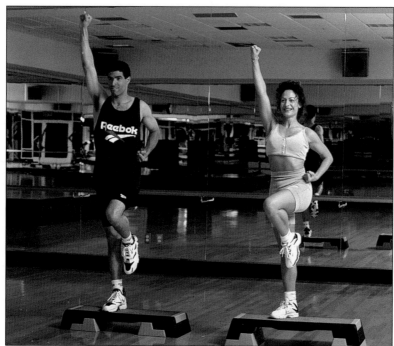

Courtesy of Step Reebok

Step aerobics is a great way to keep fit for men and women.

Why Step?

Stepping has a lot going for it. Step training requires an initial investment of a good pair of stepping shoes and a step platform, but nothing else. The simple movement routines can be accomplished by everyone, unlike some other modes of training. It also requires less space than other exercise programs available.

Consider the strengths of step training:

- **Simplicity.** Whether you choose to step in a club or at home, step movements are easy to learn and simple to execute.
- **Efficiency.** Step exercise expends the same amount of energy as walking at 4 miles per hour, jogging at 5 to 7 miles per hour, cycling at 10 to 15 miles per hour, or participating in a moderate to high intensity aerobics dance class. Although the exact energy costs depend primarily on step height, speed of stepping, individual body weight, and stepping intensity, stepping is an efficient training mode.
- **Universality.** Whether you're male or female, young or old, stepping can work for you. Special step aerobics programs have been created for young people, seniors, pre- and postnatal women, and athletes.
- **Compactness.** Stepping does require that each participant have a step platform, but most step platforms are lightweight, adjustable, and compact. Minimal assembly is required, and storage is a breeze. Step platforms can fit easily under a bed, in a closet, or be stored near a wall, and they do not require much floor space.
- **Versatility.** Step aerobics can be done on land, in the water, in your home, club, hotel room, or outdoors. It can provide you with a cardiovascular, strengthening, or flexibility workout.
- **Fun.** Step aerobics is fun. Ask any of the seven million participants who regularly flock to step aerobics classes or work out at home. The music is motivating, the steps are easy, the workout is fun, and the results are great!

As with any fitness method, step aerobics has a few hurdles you'll want to overcome:

- **Cost.** Stepping isn't a free activity unless you use the stairs in your home, but doing that is very limiting. The costs of participating in step aerobics include $20 to $80 for a step platform and between $50 and $100 for a good pair of step training shoes. The good news is that these costs are incurred only when you begin the program. Joining a club that offers step aerobics can cost from $20 to $50 a month. Single step classes can cost from $5 to $15 per class.

- **Imbalances.**   Stepping is not a complete exercise program because it specifically uses and develops the anterior (front) thigh, leg, and hip muscles. Training imbalances raise the risk of injury, so stepping needs to be combined with other strengthening and flexibility exercises.

See chapter 5 for some recommended exercises to help round out your program.

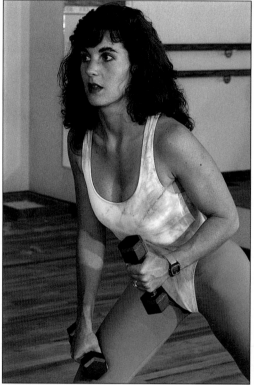

© F-Stock/David Stoechlein

To avoid training imbalances, it's best to combine stepping with other strengthening and stretching exercises.

The FITT Principle

Training sessions should be planned according to the FITT principle to achieve the greatest benefits from exercise. The FITT principle is an acronym for **F**requency of exercise, **I**ntensity of exercise, **T**ime or duration of the exercise session, and the **T**ype of exercise. Base your exercise program on these four key principles.

Frequency refers to the number of training sessions per week. Experts recommend that individuals try to exercise three to five days per week. The exact frequency is determined by the type of exercise performed, your fitness status, and your goals. Keep in mind, however, that something is always better than nothing.

Intensity refers to the level of physiologic stress attained during the exercise period. Exercise sessions can be low or high intensity. Intensity is sometimes measured by heart rate. Your heart rate during low intensity exercise would be approximately 50 to 60 percent of your maximal heart rate. Your heart rate would be approximately 85 to 90 percent of your maximal during high intensity exercise. (Maximal heart rate can be estimated by subtracting your age from 220.) In this book, we'll be using a method of measuring intensity called "perceived exertion." More on this can be found on page 56. When beginning an exercise program, it is best to start out at a low intensity and gradually increase the intensity over time.

Time refers to the duration of the training session. Duration and intensity are inversely related; if the intensity of the exercise is high, the duration is generally low, and vice versa. Thirty to 40 minutes of continuous aerobic exercise is recommended per exercise session. You must add time for flexibility and muscular training if you want a well-rounded program.

Type refers to the kind of activity performed during the exercise session. Different kinds of exercise affect fitness in different ways. For example, aerobic exercise primarily affects aerobic capacity and body composition, but it has less effect on muscular strength and flexibility.

Another important component of any exercise program is the rate of progression. *Rate of progression* refers to how fast an individual increases intensity, duration, and frequency. Rate of progression is directly related to a range of factors, including fatigue and dropout rate. That is, the faster the rate of progression, the greater the fatigue and probability of dropping out. The intensity, duration, and frequency should all be gradually increased over time—over weeks or months, not days.

Benefits of Stepping

The benefits of regular physical activity and exercise, including stepping, are becoming increasingly clearer. Individuals that choose to be more physically active in their leisure and work activities lower their risk for developing diseases such as osteoporosis, diabetes, obesity, and cardio-vascular disease in addition to sleeping better, having more energy, and just feeling great!

A simple definition of health-related physical fitness is "the ability of the body's systems (heart, lungs, blood vessels, muscles) to function effi-ciently, as to resist disease and to be able to participate in a wide variety of activities without undue fatigue." A comprehensive fitness program should have activities that develop and maintain each of the five fitness components: cardiovascular fitness, muscular strength, muscular endurance, flexibility, and body composition. The stepping program in this book is excellent because it develops all five.

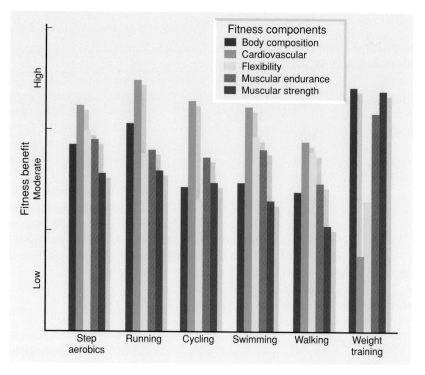

How step aerobics compares to other fitness activities.

For example, in the Green and Blue workouts, you'll get seven workouts that focus on cardiovascular fitness and three workouts that focus on muscle strengthening. All 10 workouts incorporate muscular endurance and flexibility and can improve your body composition as long as you aren't taking in excessive calories each day. Each color zone is designed to incorporate each of the fitness components in a unique way to give you a progressive challenge that will allow you to reach your personal goals. If you're more interested in cardiovascular fitness than strength, you can easily choose those workouts that will emphasize that component; however, we do recommend a balance among all five components.

ASSESSING YOUR PHYSICAL READINESS

Step aerobics can be a strenuous physical activity, especially if it's been a while since you've taken part in a physical fitness program. Seven questions from the Physical Activity Readiness Questionnaire (PAR-Q) will help you assess your readiness to start stepping. (See chapter 3 for a further assessment of your health and fitness levels.)

PAR-Q & YOU

	YES	NO
1. Has your doctor ever said that you have a heart condition *and* that you should only do physical activity recommended by a doctor?	___	___
2. Do you feel pain in your chest when you do physical activity?	___	___
3. In the past month, have you had chest pain when you were not doing physical activity?	___	___
4. Do you lose your balance because of dizziness or do you ever lose consciousness?	___	___
5. Do you have a bone or joint problem that could be made worse by a change in your physical activity?	___	___
6. Is your doctor currently prescribing drugs (for example, water pills) for your blood pressure or heart condition?	___	___
7. Do you know of *any other reason* why you should not do physical activity?	___	___

If you answer yes to any question, go no further until you receive a doctor's clearance. If you answer no to every question, you can be reasonably sure it's safe to increase your physical activity.

2

Getting Equipped

Now that we've covered some of the basics of step exercise, let's turn our attention to the specific equipment needs. Every sport or mode of exercise requires some specialized gear. Step exercise is no exception. Although it does require a bit more equipment than walking or running, it needs less than skating or biking. This chapter provides you with an overview of your equipment needs from the bare bones to the elaborate.

Depending on your tastes, you can dress with fashionably coordinated attire from head to toe, or you can be just as comfortable in a pair of baggy sweats and a T-shirt. You can spend hundreds of dollars on the most sophisticated and coordinated gear, or invest less money and purchase functional products at discounted and closeout prices. Whichever style suits your fancy, the bottom line depends on your budget and your desire for fashion.

Clothing

No matter how you choose to outfit yourself, look for the following when accumulating your workout wardrobe:

- Underwear that supports without binding

- Socks that fit snugly without bunching up in your shoes. Bunching can cause blisters.
- Shorts or sweats that allow free movement and don't irritate your inner thighs
- A variety of shirts (T-shirts, tank tops, jerseys, short- and long-sleeved shirts, or sweat shirts)
- Tights or leotards that are comfortable and nonrestricting
- Water bottle and towel
- Headband to prevent sweat from dripping onto your step

Shoes

You need special shoes for stepping because step exercisers have additional stresses placed on the Achilles tendon and the calf. A suitable shoe has good forefoot flexibility (it bends easily behind the toes) and an adequate heel lift to accommodate the stresses of step training. Step shoes or cross-training shoes made by reputable athletic shoe companies offer great forefoot cushioning and flexibility and, due to their wider heels, greater foot stability.

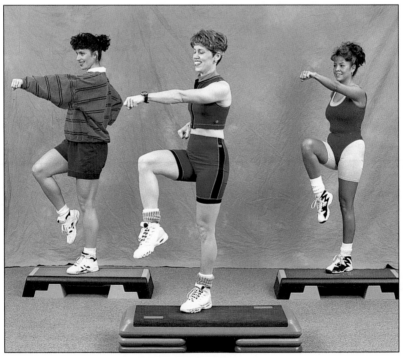

Let your budget and your taste for fashion dictate your stepping attire.

Good shoes cost between $50 and $100. Although you may find imitation brand footwear for under $50, you'll often sacrifice the essential features and durability of a well-made shoe. You can also spend more than $100, but you're probably paying for a lot more than you need.

It's a good idea to stick with reputable athletic shoe companies when making your shoe investment. *IDEA Today* and *Shape* magazines consider these companies worthy of including in their annual shoe survey: Asics, Avia, Nike, Reebok, Ryka, and Saucony.

For specific shoe recommendations, check the annual reviews in *Shape* magazine. If you have friends who work out regularly or are fitness professionals, ask them which shoe they prefer and why. No matter what their recommendation though, the best shoe for you is the one that fits best. When you've finished your research, go to a sporting goods or athletic footwear store whose staff is trained to help you make the right selection. Wear a pair of athletic socks, try on the shoes, and simulate the up-and-down stepping motion of your workout. Pay particular attention to how your feet feel during the movement. The shoe should feel snug, yet comfortable. Your toes should be able to move easily, and your heel should sit firmly in the shoe and not slide up and down.

Realize that there is no one perfect shoe. We all have individual needs due to the large variance in foot shape and size. Focus less on the new flashy colorful designs and more on support, function, and fit to choose the right shoe for you. Remember, the best advice for shoe buying is to invest in the one that fits!

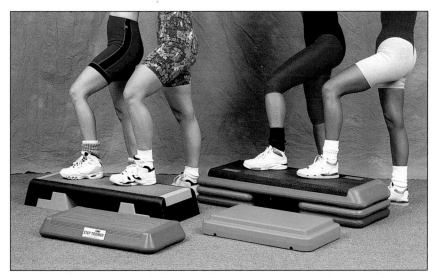

Steps, like shoes, come in all shapes and sizes; let your needs determine the step you choose.

Steps

A number of different types and brands of step platforms are available. Although the proliferation of brands may seem overwhelming, the wide selection gives you the opportunity to find the step equipment that will work best for you. Steps range in price from $15 to $80, and they can be made of a number of different materials. Solid wood steps, although usually less expensive ($15 to $20), are heavy and not adjustable. Steps made from foam are lightweight, moderately priced ($20 to $30), and usually adjustable, but they may become uncomfortable to use as the foam wears down from repeated use. Polyurethane and maple spring steps are a bit pricey (from $60 to $80), but they absorb shock and allow you to execute power moves easily. These steps are not adjustable in height. The most common step purchase is molded plastic. These relatively inexpensive steps ($20 to $25 for generic brands, or $40 to $70 for brand names) are usually adjustable, durable, lightweight, and portable. Most steps are from two to four feet long. Two-foot-long steps require less space, but they limit your ability to maneuver up, over, and around them. A four-foot-long step takes up more floor space but allows you greater room to travel. Your decision depends on what you like. Keep these and the following items in mind as you decide which step is right for you:

- **Space accommodation**. Step platforms vary in size from two to four feet long. Determine the area you'll be stepping in and make sure you have enough room for the step, as well as enough open space around the step. You should clear approximately three feet behind and in front of your step and about two feet off either end.
- **Storage**. Most steps are small and portable for easy storage in a closet or under a bed. Make sure you've thought of the storage space you need for your step platform before you make your purchase.
- **Safety**. Check the step for sturdy construction and stability. Step on it to see if you slip or if the step has a poor design.
- **Adjustability**. Can the step height be adjusted? Varying step heights provide you the option of varying workout intensity.
- **Maintenance**. How often, if at all, does the step need to be cleaned or repaired? What is its consumer satisfaction ratings? Are the joints, hardware, and top surface well constructed? How can it be repaired?
- **Guarantees**. Check for a guarantee that covers the life of the step. Does the manufacturer give an estimate of how long its product will last? Can you return the product if you're not satisfied?
- **Price comparison**. Shop around. Many outlet and discount stores have special sales on brand name products.

Ideally, you should step up and down on the platform before making your investment. Local sporting goods stores and discount department store chains carry a wide variety of step platforms to choose from. Many are on display and available for testing. We discourage ordering a step product through mail order or home shopping clubs unless you can return it for a full refund if you are dissatisfied.

Music

One of the most vital components of your step workout is your music selection. The music should be personally motivating, but it should also have a rhythm appropriate for fitness stepping. Research has shown that for safety reasons, the music beats per minute (BPM) should fall between 118 and 125, with an average around 120 BPM. Stepping to music that is too fast can significantly increase your risk of injury.

To assess the BPM of your favorite tunes, use the following simple technique. You'll need a watch with a sweep second hand or a stopwatch.

1. Play an excerpt from your music selection.
2. Tap out the beat.
3. Count how many beats you hear in six seconds.
4. Add a zero to this number. For example, if you counted 12 beats in 6 seconds, adding a zero to the count would equal 120. This gives you an estimate of the beats per minute of this selection.

You also have the option to choose premixed step aerobics music tapes from one of the fitness music companies. Some of the well known companies are Power Productions (1-800-777-BEAT), Dynamix (1-800-THE-MIXX), and Muscle Mixes (1-800-52-MIXES). Other premixed fitness music can be purchased at your local music store.

Adding Up the Costs

You can invest an enormous amount of money in clothes and equipment, or you can be frugal and spend significantly less. Let's examine a sample cost comparison, starting with the bare necessities. Then we'll look at high-end purchases.

Low-Budget Shopping

Your shopping list must contain shoes and a step platform. Choose good supportive shoes, specifically designed for stepping or cross training, from one of the major athletic footwear companies mentioned in this chapter. Look for discounted sales and bargain closeout models. You'll easily be able to find a pair for under $60. Check local stores for discounted sales on step platforms as well. Remember to check the platform for safety and stability before you make your purchase. Many retailers sell discounted step platforms for as low as $20. Dress in nonrestrictive clothing you already own and play music from your favorite collection.

LOW-BUDGET COSTS	
STEP OR CROSS-TRAINING SHOES	$50
STEP PLATFORM ON SALE	$20
TOTAL COST	$70

High-Budget Shopping

Splurge on high-end fashion shoes and matching gear. You may want two pairs of shoes (one offering more support and cushioning) to alternate from easy to hard workouts. You can buy music specifically designed for step aerobics. You can choose from rock, hip hop, country, broadway, oldies, Motown, and many others. Most tapes produced by fitness music companies are perfectly mixed, without any breaks between songs, and they follow the recommended beats per minute guidelines for step exercise.

Instead of monitoring your heart rate manually, you can invest in a heart rate monitor. They are available at sporting goods stores. They'll range in price from $100 to $200.

The following price samples aren't the highest you can go. You can add accessories such as headsets, leg warmers, water bottles, towels, workout logs, and much more.

HIGH-BUDGET COSTS	
TWO PAIRS STEP OR CROSS-TRAINING SHOES	$150
SHORTS OR TIGHTS	$30
T-SHIRT OR LEOTARD	$30
STEP (HIGH PRICE)	$70
COVER-UP OR SWEATSHIRT	$30
HEART RATE MONITOR	$100
TWO MUSIC TAPES	$50
TOTAL COST	$460

Where to Step

Plush health clubs or spas with top-notch step aerobics equipment and instructors are nice, but not necessary. Community centers, YMCAs, church halls, and your own home are all fine places for a step workout.

You can step anywhere, anytime, regardless of the weather. Step is primarily an indoor activity, although you could venture outdoors if you wanted to. Step platforms are some of the most versatile, portable, and easy-to-use props available. No matter where you choose to step, remember to equip yourself according to the guidelines given in this chapter to guarantee the safest, most productive, and enjoyable workout.

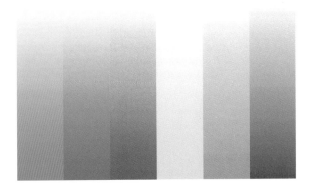

3

Assessing Your Readiness to Begin

Essential elements of good health include being relatively free from symptoms of disease and pain, being able to be active, and being in good spirits most of the time. Individuals that choose to exercise and lead active lifestyles generally enjoy better health compared to under-active individuals. In fact, scientific studies have found that 7 of the 10 leading causes of death can be substantially reduced by controlling blood pressure and stress, quitting cigarette smoking, eating wisely, getting plenty of exercise, and drinking alcohol in moderation, if at all. However, before beginning an exercise program, it is important to consider several factors, such as your present and past health status, your present fitness level, your current lifestyle, and any medical or health problems that may restrict your exercise program. The purpose of this chapter is to help you assess your readiness to begin an exercise program.

Exercise is quite safe for most individuals. Problems arise when people who have a high-risk medical or health condition start an exercise program. As these previously under-active people begin to increase their physical activity, the risk of injury resulting from exercise goes up. Before starting a step aerobics program, you need to make sure you do not have any medical or health conditions that could affect the safety and effectiveness of your exercise program. One of the most important factors to consider before you start an exercise program is whether or not the benefits of an exercise program outweigh any potential risks. Some medical and health conditions make exercise inappropriate, such as heart-related problems, severe emotional distress, alcoholism, eating disorders, orthopedic problems, recent illness or infection, breathing problems, or an extreme under-active lifestyle.

The American College of Sports Medicine recommends that men younger than 40 and women younger than 50 can start a moderate exercise program without a medical exam or exercise test if they are apparently healthy. An apparently healthy individual is defined as someone with one or fewer major coronary risk factors (table 3.1). A moderate exercise program is one where the exercise intensity is well within the individual's comfort level and can be sustained for 20 minutes or more. The program is usually noncompetitive and slow to moderate in pace.

Table 3.1
Major Coronary Risk Factors

1. Diagnosed hypertension or systolic blood pressure greater than 160 mmHg or diastolic blood pressure greater than 90 mmHg on at least two separate occasions, or on high blood pressure medication.
2. Blood cholesterol greater than 240 mg/dl
3. Cigarette smoking
4. Diabetes
5. Family history of heart disease in parents or siblings less than 55 years old.

How Is Your Health?

The Assessing Your Stepping Fitness questionnaire in this chapter can help you determine what level of step training you should start with. If you score 20 points or more, your health and fitness level is high and you can start with the intermediate or advanced step training workouts described in this book. A score of 10 to 19 points indicates your health and fitness level are average, which means you can probably start with the intermediate workouts. A score of fewer than 10 points indicates your health and fitness level is below average, and you should start with the beginning step training workouts. If you score fewer than 10 points, or are generally inactive, you may want to consult with your physician before starting a regular program of exercise. If after you start your exercise program you notice musculoskeletal soreness or pain, breathing trouble, chest pain, or any other unusual symptoms, you should stop your stepping program and consult with a physician before continuing.

ASSESSING YOUR STEPPING FITNESS

Cardiovascular Health

Which of these statements best describes your cardiovascular condition? This is a critical safety check before you enter any vigorous activity. (*Warning:* If you have a history of cardiovascular disease, start the stepping programs in this book only after receiving clearance from your doctor—and then only with close supervision by a fitness professional.)

No history of heart or circulatory problems	_____ (3)
Past ailments have been treated successfully	_____ (2)
Such problems exist but no treatment required	_____ (1)
Under medical care for cardiovascular illness	_____ (0)

Injuries

Which of these statements best describes your current injuries? This is a test of your musculoskeletal readiness to start a stepping program. (*Warning:* If your injury is temporary, wait until it is cured before starting the program. If it is chronic, adjust the program to fit your limitations.)

No current injury problems	_____ (3)
Some pain in activity but not limited by it	_____ (2)
Level of activity is limited by the injury	_____ (1)
Unable to do much strenuous training	_____ (0)

Illnesses

Which of these statements best describes your current illnesses? Certain temporary or chronic conditions will delay or disrupt your stepping program. (See warning under "Injuries.")

No current illness problems	_____ (3)
Some problem in activity but not limited by it	_____ (2)
Level of activity is limited by the illness	_____ (1)
Unable to do much strenuous training	_____ (0)

(continued)

ASSESSING YOUR STEPPING FITNESS *(continued)*

Age

Which of these age groups describes you?

Age 19 and younger	_____ (3)
Ages 20 to 29	_____ (2)
Ages 30 to 39	_____ (1)
Ages 40 and older	_____ (0)

Weight

Which of these figures best describes how close you are to your own definition of "ideal weight"? Excess fat can be a major mark of unfitness, but it's also possible to be significantly underweight.

Within 5 pounds of ideal weight	_____ (3)
6 to 10 pounds above or below the ideal	_____ (2)
11 to 19 pounds above or below ideal weight	_____ (1)
20 or more pounds above or below the ideal	_____ (0)

Resting Pulse Rate

Which of these figures describes your current pulse rate on waking up but before getting out of bed? A well-trained heart beats slower and more efficiently than one that's unfit.

Below 60 beats per minute	_____ (3)
60 to 69 beats per minute	_____ (2)
70 to 79 beats per minute	_____ (1)
80 or more beats per minute	_____ (0)

Smoking

Which of these statements best describes your smoking history and current habit (if any)? Smoking is a major enemy of health and fitness.

Never a smoker	_____ (3)
Once a smoker but quit	_____ (2)
An occasional, light smoker now	_____ (1)
A regular, heavy smoker now	_____ (0)

Most Recent Group Aerobic Workout

Which of these statements best describes your group aerobic exercise schedule within the last month? A good way to tell your readiness for stepping is your level of involvement in group aerobics.

Participate in aerobic exercise classes more than
3 times a week   _____ (3)

Participate in aerobic exercise classes 2 to 3 times
a week   _____ (2)

Participate in aerobic exercise classes 1 to 2 times
a week   _____ (1)

No recent aerobic exercise classes   _____ (0)

Aerobic Exercise Background

Which of these statements best describes your aerobic step exercise history? Stepping fitness isn't long-lasting, but the fact that you once stepped is a good sign that you can do it again.

Participated in aerobic step workouts 1 to 2 years ago   _____ (3)

Participated seriously on a regular basis within the
past year   _____ (2)

Participate in aerobic step workouts 1 to 2 times a week   _____ (1)

No recent aerobic step training   _____ (0)

Related Activities

Which of these statements best describes your participation in other exercises that are similar to stepping in their aerobic benefit such as running, walking, biking, or swimming?

Regularly practice similar aerobic activities   _____ (3)

Regularly practice less vigorous aerobic activities   _____ (2)

Regularly practice nonaerobic sports (weightlifting,
tennis, golf)   _____ (1)

Not regularly active in any physical activities   _____ (0)

Total score _____

Reprinted, by permission, from R.L. Brown and J. Henderson, 1994, *Fitness Running* (Champaign, IL: Human Kinetics), 22-25.

Test Your Stepping Fitness

It is important to know your aerobic capacity (cardiovascular endurance) before you plan your step training program. The STEP Fit Test, designed by Dr. James Rippe, lets you find this. The only equipment needed to perform the test is an 8-inch step, a stopwatch or a watch with a second hand, and a metronome or piece of music with a rhythm of 76 beats per minute. The test is made up of two assessments: heart rate measurement and physical activity level. Your fitness category will be determined by correlating these two figures.

Taking the STEP Fit Test

Before you try to take the STEP Fit Test, you need to be able to accurately take your heart rate. Place the index, middle, and ring finger of one hand on the inner wrist of your other hand, just below the wrist bone and directly down from the base of the thumb. Count each pulse beat that you feel for six seconds. Multiply your count by 10 to get your heart rate per minute.

Take a few minutes to warm up before you begin the test. You might want to do a warm-up by walking at a moderate pace for 5 to 10 minutes. Some light stretching might also be beneficial (see chapter 5). The test is really quite simple. All you need to do is step up and down on an 8-inch step using a 4-count sequence (right foot up on the platform, left foot up on the platform, right foot down on the floor, left foot down on the floor). The stepping must be conducted at a cadence of 76 counts per minute. After three minutes of stepping, stop and *immediately* count your pulse rate.

Finding Your Fitness Category

First, complete the Current Physical Activity Level questionnaire to determine your current level of physical activity. After you complete the questionnaire, find the Relative Fitness Levels chart for your age and gender. Next, find your one-minute heart rate (the one you took at the end of the STEP Fit Test) on the left side of the chart and your current activity level at the bottom of the chart.

CURRENT PHYSICAL ACTIVITY LEVEL

Use the appropriate number (0-7), which best describes your general activity level for the previous month.

I do not participate regularly in programmed recreational sport or heavy physical activity.

0   I avoid walking or exertion; for example, always use the elevator, drive whenever possible instead of walking.

1   I walk for pleasure, routinely use stairs, and occasionally exercise sufficiently to cause heavy breathing or perspiration.

I participate regularly in recreation or work requiring modest physical activity, such as golf, horseback riding, calisthenics, gymnastics, table tennis, bowling, weight lifting, or yard work.

2   I exercise 10-60 minutes per week.

3   I exercise for over one hour per week.

I participate regularly in heavy physical exercise such as running or jogging, swimming, cycling, rowing, skipping rope, running in place or engaging in vigorous aerobic activity-type exercise such as tennis, basketball or handball.

4   I spend less than 30 minutes per week in physical activity, or run less than one mile per week.

5   I spend 30-60 minutes per week in physical activity, or run one mile per week.

6   I spend 1-3 hours per week in physical activity, or run 5-10 miles per week.

7   I spend over 3 hours per week in physical activity, or run over 10 miles per week.

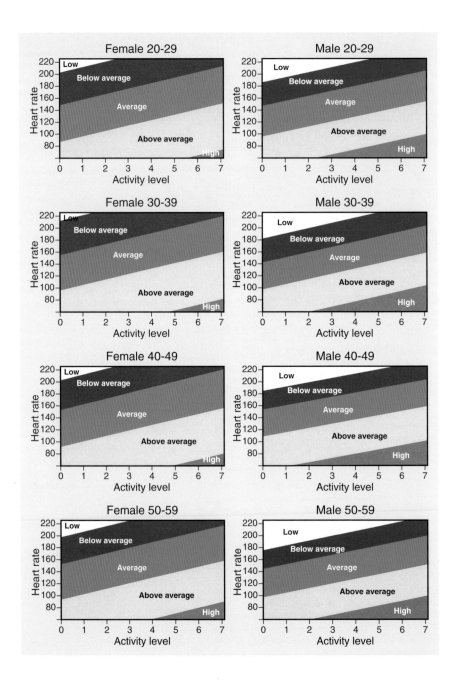

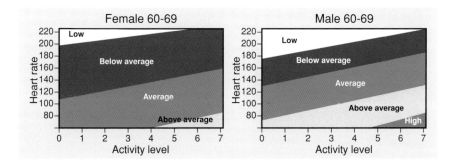

Note: These charts were designed for fitness stepping specifically, not for general fitness. Use them as guidelines only to give you an idea of your present level of aerobic fitness.

FITNESS STEPPING, © 1993, the STEP Company. Relative Fitness Levels are reproduced with permission. For a complete FITNESS STEPPING brochure with the STEP FIT test and Fitness Testing Prescriptions please send a self-addressed, stamped envelope to the STEP Company, 2250 New Market Parkway, Suite 130, Marietta, GA 30067

After you have located your heart rate and current physical activity level, draw a vertical line through your activity level and a horizontal line through your heart rate. The point where the lines intersect is your fitness level as determined by the American Heart Association standards. You can record this data in your Personal Fitness Assessment Summary Chart below.

PERSONAL FITNESS ASSESSMENT SUMMARY CHART					
Date					
One-minute heart rate (after test)					
Current physical activity level (0-7)					
Relative fitness level (high . . . low)					
Color-coded workout zone (Green-Red)					

The STEP Fit Test was designed to estimate your aerobic capacity. It is not as accurate as a direct measurement of aerobic capacity in a laboratory setting. However, the charts are a good way to assess how fit you are compared to other individuals of your age and gender. Every six months to one year, you should take the STEP Fit Test to assess changes in your fitness level. As your fitness level improves, you will need to advance to more difficult stepping programs if you want to continue to improve your aerobic capacity.

If after you finish the STEP Fit Test you fall into a low fitness category (low or below average), it is advisable that you start off with a beginning step aerobics workout program (Green or Blue zones). If you fall into a higher fitness category (average or above), you should start with the intermediate or advanced step aerobics workouts (Purple to Red zones). Another benefit of taking the STEP Fit Test periodically is so you can see the improvement in your fitness level.

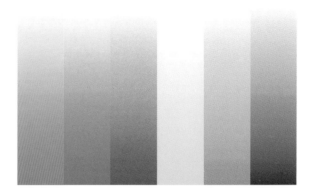

4

Stepping the Right Way

Who would ever believe that there's a right way to step up and down? We do it every day! However, taking steps as part of a daily activity is somewhat different from the varied techniques and movements used in step aerobics. Stepping is an excellent form of exercise, but it must be done correctly. So, to get the most from your step workouts and remain injury free, follow the guidelines and techniques presented in this chapter.

Body Alignment

An important starting point for safe stepping is good postural alignment. The basic postural position is the same for all steppers. However, because of the differences in body shapes and sizes, the way you'll look once you've aligned yourself may differ from other people.

A *neutral posture* will reduce excessive stress on your spine. According to many experts, it is the safest alignment for standing, sitting, lifting, and lying. Although each individual's neutral posture may vary slightly, in general, you will have a slight inward curve at the neck and low back, and a slight outward curve of the midback. Because lower back pain afflicts approximately 80 percent of us at some time, it is important to apply a neutral posture to your stepping to help you avoid lower back pain. Use this method for checking your posture.

First, stand in front of a full-length mirror. Pay attention to your body as a whole. Now, begin at the top and work your way down. Lift your head so it is naturally extended from your spine. Avoid jutting the chin forward. Keep your shoulders down so that they are relaxed. Keeping your head and shoulders aligned, gently tighten your abdominal muscles, as if you're trying to zip up a snug pair of blue jeans. Gently rock your pelvis forward and back until you find a comfortable position that is not exaggerated in either direction.

In your profile position in front of the mirror, lock your knees and notice how that affects your posture. Did your back arch, causing your abdomen to push forward? Try to keep your knees relaxed to avoid this problem.

For the final check, focus on your feet. Naturally aligned feet have slight arches and do not roll in or out. Many knee and back problems often stem from a disorder in the feet. If your feet naturally roll out (inversion), roll in (eversion), or have no arch, a podiatrist can give you relief by prescribing a shoe insert (an orthotic) to meet your needs.

Stepping Safely

Now that you've established your naturally balanced posture, let's look at how to step the right way. It's important that you learn and use correct body mechanics for safe stepping. To progress safely and remain injury free, follow these pointers when starting your stepping program.

Step Height

Carefully select the appropriate height for your step. Novice steppers should begin on a four-inch step, while more experienced steppers can use a six- to eight-inch step. Only highly skilled athletes should use a 10-inch step. Regardless of individual step fitness levels or experience, you should not exercise with a step height that causes your knee joint to bend more than 90 degrees.

Step Security

Before you begin, make sure that your step is secure on the floor. Place one foot completely atop the step and give a slight push to make sure it won't slip, slide, or come apart. Once this safety check has been completed, you're ready to step right up.

Stepping Posture

Maintain a neutral posture with your head erect, shoulders down and back, chest uplifted, and pelvis in a neutral position. Do not lock the knees at any time. When stepping up, lean slightly forward from the ankles. Leaning from the waist or neck can place excessive stress on the lower back.

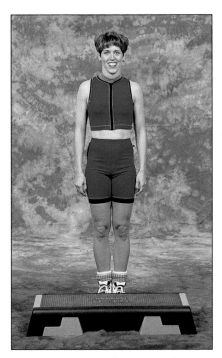 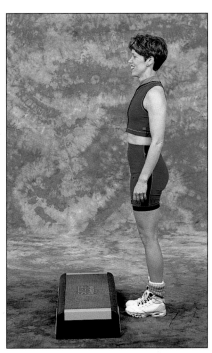

Maintaining a neutral posture is important for safe and effective stepping.

Foot Contact

The entire sole of the foot should make contact with the step platform while stepping. To avoid Achilles tendinitis (inflammation of the Achilles tendon), don't let your heels hang off the edge of the step.

Step gently onto the platform. When stepping down, step close to the platform and allow your heels to touch the floor to help absorb stress on the feet. Stepping back too far can strain the Achilles tendon area.

THE *WRONG* STEPS

Stepping Backward

Blind stepping, or stepping with your back toward the step, makes it almost impossible to be totally aware of your foot placement. Avoid blind stepping at all times.

Stepping Forward

Although we step forward off steps everyday, repeated forward stepping increases the risk of injury to the knee. Stepping forward should be limited.

Jumping onto and off of the Step

Athletes can be seen jumping onto and off of step platforms in an attempt to increase their speed and strength. In spite of the benefits these plyometric activities provide elite athletes, a relatively high risk to the feet, knees, and low back exists for the nonathlete.

Crossing the Feet While Stepping

Crossing your feet when traveling over the top of the step increases the risk of injury to the lower legs and knees and increases the risk for tripping. Don't cross your feet while stepping.

Turning Movements With a Loaded Knee

A loaded knee is one that is bearing weight. For example, when you're standing on one leg, that knee is loaded. Attempting turning step movements while bearing weight at the knee is risky. When turning, always lift the heel so the weight is on the ball of the foot. You can then pivot easily and move the limbs freely.

Stepping Speed

Music speeds from 118 to 125 beats per minute are fairly safe and common for most step workouts. See chapter 2 for an explanation of determining appropriate beats per minute of music.

No Stepping

Remember that step aerobics, when done correctly, is a great form of exercise, yet it's not for everyone. Individuals with chronic joint or back problems, women who are pregnant, people with high blood pressure, or underactive individuals over age 40 should have permission from their physicians to begin this program.

Starting Positions and Step Language

Now that you understand the foundations and safety issues related to safe stepping, we need to learn the variety of directional approach positions (pictured below) before getting into the actual basic step movements.

Step movements can begin from the *front* (the step is on the floor in front of your feet), the *side* (standing on the floor with the side of your body next to the long side of the step), the *top* (standing atop the step), the *end* (standing on the floor at the short end of the step), the *corner* (standing on the floor at one corner), and *astride* (standing on the floor and straddling the step). Refer to the illustrations and review these positions as often as needed.

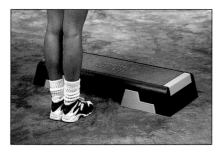

Front

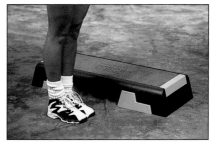

Side

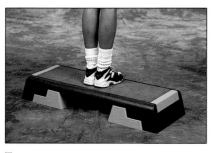

Top

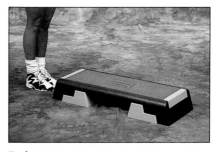

End

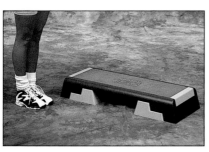

Corner

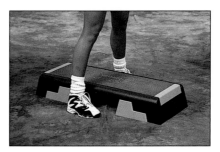

Astride

The language of step is easy because most terms refer to the exact movements you execute. For example, in a *knee up*, you step onto the platform with one foot while lifting the opposite knee. All step training movements are classified as either *single lead steps* or *alternating lead steps*. A *single right lead step* indicates that the right foot will initiate (lead) the movement each time the step pattern is repeated. An *alternating lead step* indicates that the lead foot (the foot starting the movement) will alternate between right and left each time the step pattern is repeated. Greater musculoskeletal stress is placed on the lead leg, so a single lead step should be performed for no more than one minute before changing the lead to the other foot.

Basic Foot Movements

All step training programs should begin with a thorough understanding of the basic movements. The following basic step movements are designed to give you a strong foundation from which you will build your step training program.

Basic Step Up (Single or Alternating Lead)

Starting position: Front, end, or astride

Step up onto the platform with your right foot. Now step up with your left foot. Step down with your right foot first, followed by your left. This is considered a cycle. The cadence for this step is up, up, down, down.

To change lead legs (alternating lead), simply tap the left foot down on the floor following each cycle (instead of planting it), and step up with the left foot first. The cadence for an alternating lead basic step up is up, up, down, tap.

V Step (Single or Alternating Lead)

Starting position: Front

Step onto the platform, placing your right foot toward the upper right end of the step. Now step up with your left foot toward the upper left end of the step. Your feet are now open atop the step, forming an imaginary letter V. Step down with your right foot, and then place your left down and next to your right. The cadence for the single lead V step is up, up, down, down.

For an alternating lead V step, you'll need to tap the left foot down on the floor and step up with the left foot first for the second cycle. The cadence for the alternating lead V step is up, up, down, tap.

Basic Step Down (Single or Alternating Lead)

Starting position: Top

Step down with your right foot followed by your left. Then step up with your right foot followed by your left. You will start and end this cycle on top of the step. To change lead legs, tap your left foot atop the step, and repeat the cycle with the left leg leading. The cadence for a single lead basic step down is down, down, up, up. The cadence for an alternating basic step down is down, down, up, tap.

Knee Up (Single or Alternating Lead)

Starting position: Front, side, end, or astride

Step onto the platform with your right foot. Lift your left knee up. Place your left foot back down on the floor. Tap your right foot on the floor, next to your left. Repeat. The cadence for this single lead knee up is up, knee, down, tap.

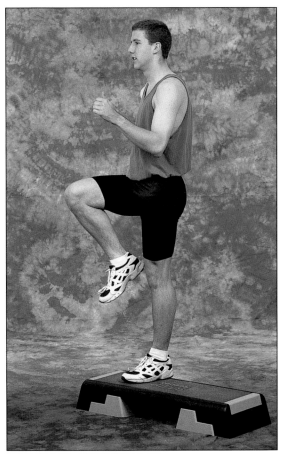

For an alternating lead, step onto the platform with your right foot. Lift your left knee up. Place your left foot back down on the floor. Put your right foot on the floor. Repeat with the left leg leading. To alternate knee ups from the side position, you need to step over and straddle the step to begin from the other side or turn your body when on the floor so the opposite lead can begin the next cycle. The cadence for the alternating knee up is up, knee, down, down; up, knee, down, down.

Tap Up and Tap Down (Single or Alternating Lead)

Starting position: Front, side, end, top, or astride

For the tap up, step up with your right foot then tap your left foot atop the step next to your right. Step down with your left foot and tap your right foot on the floor. Repeat with the same lead leg. For the tap down, begin atop the step, step down with your right foot then tap your left foot on the floor next to your right. Step up with your left foot and tap your right foot atop the step. The cadence for the single lead tap up and tap down is up, tap, down, tap or down, tap, up, tap.

For an alternating lead tap up from the front, end, or astride positions, step up with your right foot first, then tap your left foot atop the step next to your right. Step down with your left foot and step down with your right foot. Now, begin the tap ups with your left leg leading. To do an alternating lead tap down, follow the same pattern starting from atop the step, stepping down with your right foot first. The cadence for the alternating tap up and tap down step is up, tap, down, down; up, tap, down, down or down, tap, up, up; down, tap, up, up.

Power Jump Up

Starting position: Front, end, or astride

Using a two-foot takeoff, jump up onto the step. Step down with the right foot and then the left. Repeat. To provide balance to this power step, alternate step down lead legs. The cadence for the power jump up is jump up, hold, down, down. *Note.* Don't jump down; only jump up.

Power Leap Up (Single or Alternating Lead)

Starting position: Front, side, end, astride, or corner

Using a single-foot takeoff, leap onto the step with your right foot. Tap the left foot on the step next to the right. Step down with the left foot and then tap the right on the floor next to the left. Repeat. The cadence for the single lead power leap up is leap up, tap up, step down, tap down.

The alternating lead power leap up uses a single-foot leap as well. Leap up with your right foot. Tap the left foot on the step. Step down with the left foot and then step down with the right. Repeat with the left leg leading. The cadence for the alternating lead power leap up is leap up, tap, down, down; leap up, tap, down, down. *Note.* When alternating leap steps from the side starting position, you must switch to the opposite side with each alternating step. For example, right leg leap up is executed with your right side to the step. When you change to the left leg leap up, your left side would be to the side of the step.

Over the Top (Alternating Lead)

Starting position: Side

Step up to the center of the platform with your right foot. Step your left foot up next to the right. Step the right foot down on the opposite side of the step. The left foot comes off the step and taps down next to the right foot. Repeat from the beginning with the left foot, moving back up and over the top of the step, returning to your original position. The cadence for the over the top step is up (on top), up, down (on floor), over down, tap.

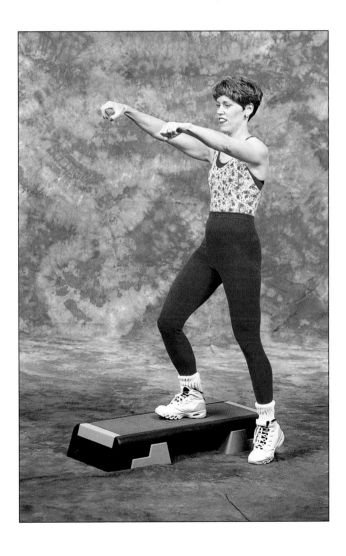

Repeater (Alternating Lead)

Starting position: Front, side, end, or astride
Step up with the right foot. Lift the left knee up. Tap the left foot down on the floor. Lift the left knee up again. Tap the left foot down on the floor. Lift the left knee up once more. Step the left foot down on the floor. Step the right foot down. Repeat from the beginning with the left leg leading. The cadence for the repeater is up, knee lift, tap down, knee lift, tap down, knee lift, step down, step down.

Straddle Up/Straddle Down (Single or Alternating Lead)

Starting position: Astride
Step up with your right foot and then your left. Straddle your right foot down, back to its original position, followed by your left. Repeat. The cadence for the single lead straddle up is up, up, down, down.

For the alternating lead straddle up, tap the left foot down on the floor and repeat the cycle with the left leg leading. The cadence for the alternating lead straddle up is up, up, down, tap; up, up, down, tap.

Straddle downs can be executed from atop the step. The cadence for single lead straddle downs is down, down, up, up. The alternating straddle downs cadence is down, down, up, tap.

Floor Movements

Marching in place, moving around the step, and tapping the feet atop the step are low impact floor moves used during the warm-ups, cool-downs, and in the step workouts to decrease the intensity of the choreography. Step touches and jumping jacks are also used in the workouts to provide variety to the step routines. To do a step touch, take one side step with the right foot then tap the left foot next to the right foot. Repeat, beginning with the left foot stepping to the left. *Note.* Executing floor movements to the beat of the music will help you maintain a consistent intensity during your workouts.

Turn Step (Alternating Lead)

Starting position: Front or side
Step up with your right foot and then your left. Step down with your right foot as you complete a one-quarter turn to the right. Tap the left foot down next to the right as your body turns. Repeat, beginning with the left leg and turning to the left. The cadence for the turn step is up, up, down & turn, tap. *Note.* Remember to unload the knee by lifting the heel and turning on the ball of the foot.

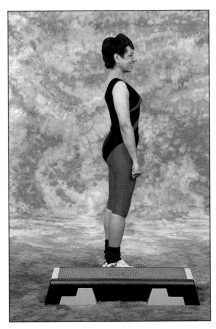

Turn step starting with side position.

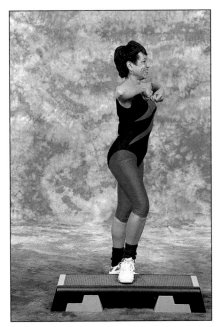

Step up with your right foot.

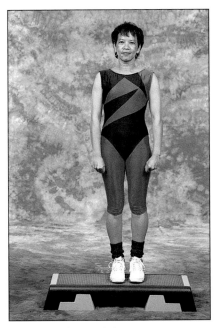

Step up with your left.

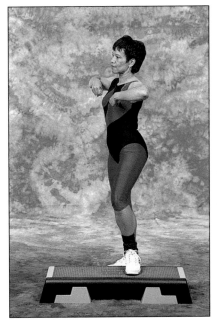

Step down with your right.

Lunge (Single or Alternating Lead)

Starting position: Top

Without shifting your body weight forward, tap down (behind) with the right foot. Then tap the right foot to the starting position. Repeat. The cadence for the single lead lunge is tap down, tap up.

For the alternating lunge, tap down with the right foot then place the right foot in the starting position. Tap down with the left foot then place the left foot in the starting position. Alternate between left and right lead legs. The cadence for the alternating lunge is tap down right, on top right, tap down left, on top left.

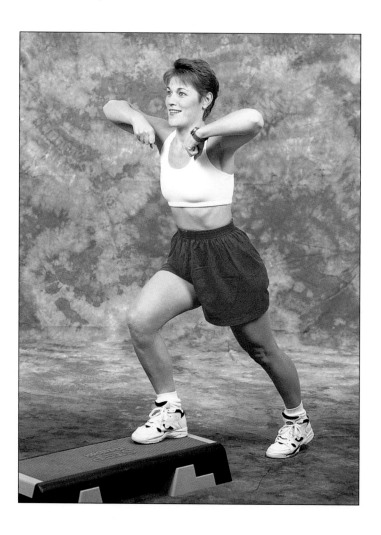

Propulsion (Power Moves)

Most basic step movements can increase in intensity when you add propulsion. By definition, *propulsion* is the act of pushing upward, forward, or ahead. In step training, propulsion moves cause the body to lift upward in an explosive yet controlled fashion. For example, adding propulsion to the over the top move would find you stepping onto the platform with the right foot, leaping into the air to land on the left foot, and stepping down off of the platform with the right foot followed by the left foot. Propulsion moves are executed upward and atop the step only.

Including propulsion, or *power moves* as they've come to be called, does not alter the cadence or count of the move. For example, in a basic step, you step up, up, down, down, using a total of four counts. In a propulsion or power basic step, your first two steps are hop or jog steps (you hop on the right foot then hop on the left foot while atop the step) and then step down, down. The move is still a total of four counts. Avoid propelling down toward the floor, because this increases your risk of injury. As you progress through this program, feel free to add these explosive movements to add greater challenges.

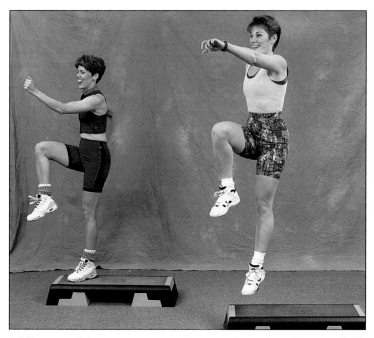

Adding propulsion to a movement increases intensity: a knee up (left) and power knee up (right).

Basic Arm Movements

You may want to start your beginning step workouts with minimal arm movements. A free-flowing arm swing, with the arms gently swinging forward and back as they do when you walk up and down stairs, should be sufficient until you get accustomed to the foot patterns and increase your endurance capabilities. When you feel ready to progress, you will need to be familiar with the following basic arm movements.

Curl Up (Biceps)

Start with both arms relaxed at the sides of your body. Without elevating your shoulders, which increases tension in the neck, bend the elbows so the palms of your hands move toward the front of your shoulders, then return to the starting position. Keep your fingers relaxed and slightly open instead of clenching your fists, which increases pressure in the forearm region.

Press Down (Triceps)

Begin with the elbows bent and the thumbs of each hand on the front of the shoulders. With an open palm, straighten the elbows, as the palms push down toward the floor. For a more challenging version, straighten the elbows as you push the palms out from the sides of the body. Pay careful attention not to lock or pop the elbow joint.

Upright Row (Deltoids)

Start with both arms relaxed and palms on the front of your thighs. Lift both arms upward, bending both elbows, as the palms approach the front of the shoulders. Return to the starting position and repeat. Make sure your shoulders stay down and relaxed.

Pull Down (Latissimus Dorsi)

Start with both arms reaching overhead. Pull both arms down, bending the elbows, so that the elbows come slightly behind the waist area. Return to the starting position and repeat.

Reach (Deltoids)

Start with arms relaxed at your sides. With straight elbows, reach your arms out in front of you. Return to the starting position and repeat. For a more challenging version, reach the arms overhead. Avoid arching the back when reaching overhead. Other variations include reaching to the side or back.

Pull Back (Trapezius)

Begin with your arms stretched out in front of your body, at shoulder height. Keeping your shoulders down and relaxed, bend both elbows as you pull your arms back and behind you, causing the shoulder blades to come together. Return to the starting position and repeat.

Fun-Time Arms

It's OK to make up your own arm movements and have some fun. Maybe you're into athletics and want to enact swinging a baseball bat or dunking a basketball. If you're into dance or stylized movements, go ahead and try the "Chicken," the "Swim," or any other movements you enjoy. Arm movements are incorporated into a step workout as a complementary or supplemental component of the workout. They help to keep the workout fun and exciting, especially if combined with your favorite music.

Wrap-Up

Fun, injury-free stepping can be attained by combining the specifics covered in this chapter with a proper warm-up before you begin and a cool-down upon completion. Because stepping primarily emphasizes the front leg muscles (the quadriceps and hip flexors), we'll place special attention on these areas as we discuss warm-ups and cool-downs.

The next chapter will deal with techniques for an effective step warm-up and cool-down.

5

Warming Up and Cooling Down

If I were to ask you what the most efficient way is to get your car running smoothly each morning, what would you tell me? I'm certain most of you would agree that starting the engine, allowing it to idle, then gradually accelerating as you drive away would be a successful strategy.

Your body, like your car, needs ample warm-up time. Warm-ups have become a common exercise term; however, your warm-up must be specific to the fitness activity you'll be engaging in to be most effective. For example, tapping the step, marching atop the step, or climbing a few flights of stairs would be components of a sensible step aerobics warm-up to accompany the traditional general warm-ups of reaching, marching in place, and so on. Stretching, which has been included as a typical warm-up activity, will be done after your workout as part of your cool-down.

Warm It Up

The warm-up segment of your workout should contain movements similar to those you'll do in the step workout. Therefore, stepping onto the platform, tapping your feet atop the step, slow stepping, and marching should be added to general, overall warm-ups.

It is up to you to notice and analyze how your body is responding to your warm-up. In addition to warming, loosening, and preparing you physically, the warm-up tests your ability to truly work out on any given day.

For example, suppose after a stressful day at the office you feel as if you have no energy to work out. Although you may truly believe you don't have the capability to work out, the few minutes you spend in the warm-up will reveal the truth. Many times, the fatigued feeling of a stressful day is overcome by a workout. After your warm-up, you'll know if you can go on or not. Most importantly, listen to your body. If it's telling you not to continue, then don't.

Ease into your workouts. Warm up for 5 to 8 minutes, roughly the length of two songs. Choose a variety of movements at a moderate pace that keeps your entire body moving, especially the lower part, since this area is the primary focus of a step workout. If you plan to incorporate arm movements like overhead reaches and curl ups in your step workout, you'll also want to include some upper body and low back warm-ups. Shoulder circles, gentle arm reaches, and back arch ups or "cat stretches" can be done in your warm-ups.

At this point you may begin to sweat. The warm-up should not cause you to be breathless. You should be able to speak effortlessly, and your breathing pattern should be comfortable.

Cool It Down

The cool-down phase of your workout is just as important as the warm-up phase. You wouldn't turn off your car abruptly when it's running at 55 miles per hour, and you shouldn't stop immediately after a heart-pumping step workout. Your cool-down should contain the same movements as your warm-up, but it should be performed at a decreasing intensity. For example, at the beginning of the cool-down, you may stop all arm movements, return to a basic step movement, and eventually work into a march on the floor or a tap on your step. Allow approximately five minutes for your stepping cool-down.

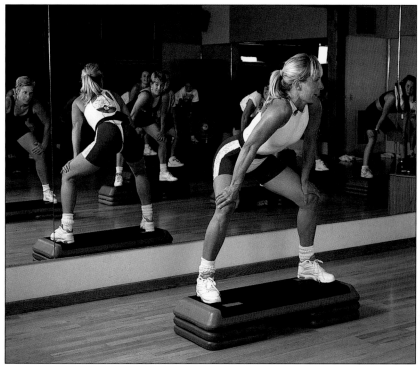

© F-Stock/Kirk Andersen

Strengthening and stretching exercises should be part of evey cool-down.

Stepping emphasizes the anterior (front) leg muscles and can reduce flexibility there. It can also cause muscle imbalances between the quadriceps and hamstring muscles if you don't exercise other parts of the leg, back, and abdomen. We recommend that you do strengthening and stretching exercises at the end of the stepping cool-down period. Some good strengthening and stretching exercises are described on pages 48 through 54.

Do the strengthening exercises first, and then the stretches to counteract the imbalanced muscle usage that occurred during your step workout and to return your body to its pre-exercise state. Don't abruptly stop exercising and sit down. Keep moving. Gradually allow your heart rate and breathing to return to normal. Pay careful attention to how your body feels, and take as much time as you need. On average, spend 5 to 10 minutes strengthening and 5 to 7 minutes stretching.

Strengthening and Stretching Exercises

The remainder of this chapter illustrates strengthening and stretching exercises that you can use to maintain and enhance muscular strength, balance, and flexibility. Strengthening and stretching your muscles needs to be slow and deliberate. Moving too quickly or haphazardly can result in injury. Be totally focused and concentrate on each part of your body during each strengthening and stretching exercise.

Strengthening and Stretching Pointers

Pay attention to the following pointers for strengthening and stretching:

Speed

- Execute strengthening exercises slowly and through a full range of motion. When stretching, do so slowly and gradually. Do not bounce or stretch to the point of pain.
- Find the initial point of discomfort (tightness). Stretch to, *not beyond*, this point.

Breathing

- Breathe normally and comfortably. Don't hold your breath. Exhale on the exertion, inhale on the relaxation during strengthening exercises.

Length of time

- Hold each stretch for 10 to 30 seconds or longer.

Muscle fatigue

- Exercise to the point of muscle fatigue, not muscle failure. A slight tingle in the working muscles is a good indication they are fatigued.

Strengthening Exercises

If you are new to an exercise program, or if you have been away from one for some time, you need to start slowly. Beginners can attempt one set of 12 repetitions for each of the following strengthening exercises. For more experienced exercisers, two to three sets of 12 repetitions should be done.

Abdominal Curl

Lie on your back with your feet resting on your step. Contract your abdominals to place your body in neutral posture. Exhale while raising your shoulder blades off the floor. Curl up as you reach toward your step. Hold briefly, and slowly lower down. Keep your head and neck in neutral position. Avoid jutting your chin forward. You may place your hands anywhere that is comfortable.

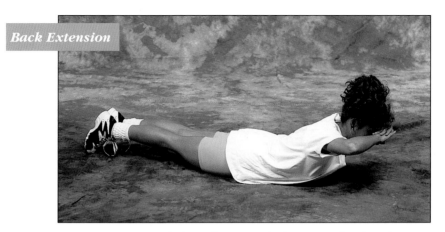

Back Extension

Lie on your abdomen. Bend your elbows and place your forehead on top of your hands. While keeping your forehead and hands in contact with each other, raise your upper body to your comfort point. Hold and breathe comfortably. Return to starting position and repeat.

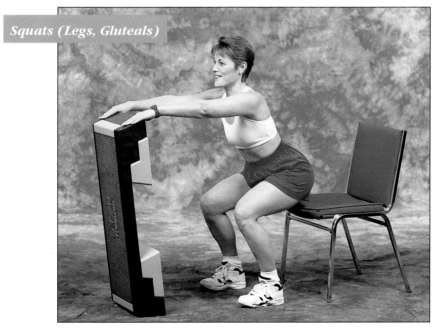

Squats (Legs, Gluteals)

Place the step upright on its end and stand a comfortable distance from a chair while holding onto your step in front of you. Slowly lower yourself toward the chair. Before making contact with the chair, return to standing position. Repeat.

Note. If your knees bother you, don't squat down so low.

Single Leg Lunge (Quadriceps, Hamstrings, Gluteals)

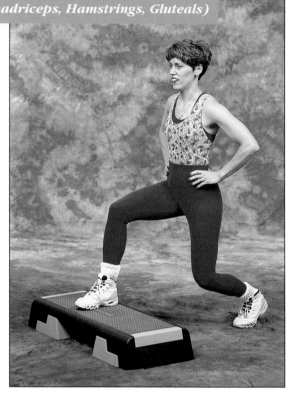

With your right foot atop the step and your left foot firmly planted on the floor behind your step, bend your knees as you lower your body down. Your front knee should be directly above your ankle. Avoid shifting your body weight forward or back, which places additional stress on the knee joints. Don't bend your knees past 90 degrees. If you suffer from knee pain, you may choose not to bend even that low. Squeeze the thigh and buttock muscles as you return to the starting position. You may alternate legs with every repetition or choose to do an entire set (12 repetitions on each leg) before switching.

Stretching Exercises

Beginners should attempt one set of the following stretches, holding each stretch for approximately 10 to 30 seconds. Experienced stretchers should do two or three sets of all the stretches, holding each stretch for 30 to 40 seconds.

Calf Stretch (Gastrocnemius and Soleus)

Stand on your step. With straight legs, gently lower your right heel off the back of your step. Hold and breathe comfortably. Keep your leg straight, but not locked. Now gently bend your right knee to deepen the stretch. Hold and breathe comfortably. Repeat with the left leg.

Front Lower Leg (Anterior Tibialis)

Stand on your step. Place the shoelaces of your right shoe on the back side of your step. Gently push the top of your foot into the step. You'll feel a stretch up the front of your foot and lower leg. Hold and breathe comfortably. Repeat with your other foot.

Upper Thigh (Hip Flexor)

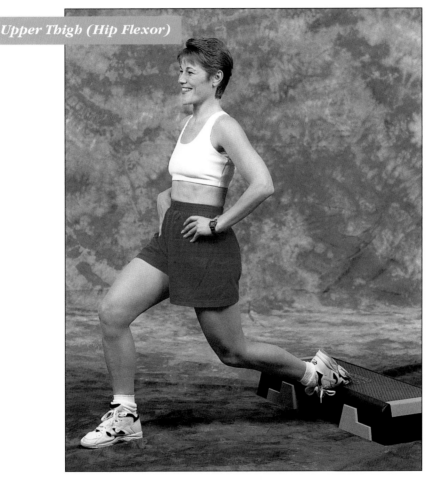

Stand on your step. Step down and forward with your right foot. Keep your feet a comfortable distance apart so you feel stable. With your left knee directly below your left hip, place your left palm on your left hip bone. Gently press your left hip bone into the palm of your hand. Gently bend your left knee. Hold and breathe comfortably. Repeat on the other leg.

Back Thigh and Buttocks (Hamstrings and Gluteals)

Standing behind your step, place your right heel on your step. Keeping your right leg straight, bend at your torso. Place your hands on your upper left thigh for support. Hold the stretch and breathe comfortably. For a deeper stretch tilt your tailbone upward and to the rear.

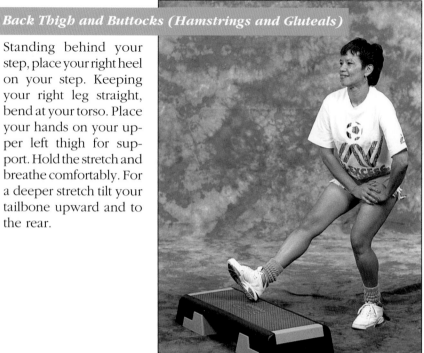

Hamstring Stretch

Sit on the floor with both legs extended in front of you. Keep your torso upright and your spine in a neutral position. Bend your right knee and slide the heel in toward your upper left thigh. Wrap a towel under the arch of your left

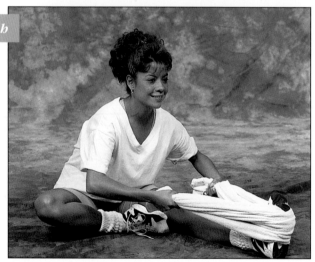

shoe. Bend at the waist while holding onto the towel and tilting the tailbone upward and toward the rear. Hold and breathe comfortably.

Quadriceps Stretch

Stand with your feet together and your torso in a neutral position. Remember that in a neutral position your head and neck are upright and slightly drawn in as a natural extension of your spine, your abdomen is held in firmly, and you have a natural curvature in your low back. Hold onto a chair, your step, or a wall for balance. Gently bend one leg, keeping the knees together. Hold onto the ankle region of the bent leg. Hold and breathe comfortably. *Note.* If this stretch causes you pain, or if you suffer from knee joint problems, place a towel around the ankle of the stretching leg. Instead of holding onto the ankle region, hold onto the ends of the towel. This will decrease the amount of flexion (bending) in your knee, yet will allow you to accomplish the stretch.

Lower Back (Erector Spinae)

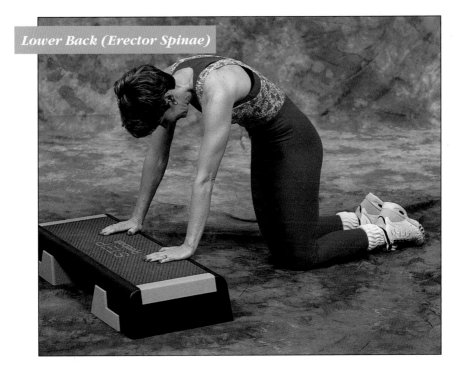

Kneeling behind your step, place your hands on top of your step. Arch your back upward while pushing your tailbone downward. Hold and breathe comfortably. Return to the starting position and repeat.

Neck and Arms

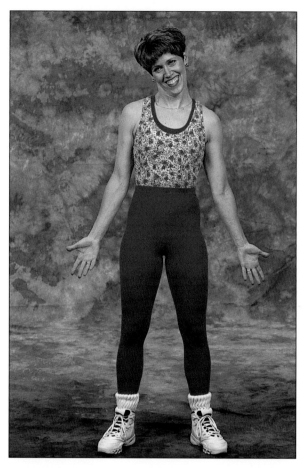

Stand with both arms at your side. Maintain a neutral posture. Reach your fingers toward the floor with the palms facing forward. Tilt your head toward your right shoulder while reaching further with your left palm. Repeat, tilting the head toward the left shoulder while reaching further with your right palm.

Summary

In this section you've learned specific strengthening and stretching exercises that will complement your step workout. To achieve maximum results from your program, we strongly recommend you always allow time for strengthening and stretching activities. You won't regret the extra time you spend!

Now that we've reviewed what to do before and after your step workout, read on for the suggested workouts.

PART II

STEP WORKOUT ZONES

This book takes a unique approach to categorizing workouts. The workouts are divided into color-coded zones according to each workout's movement selection, duration, and intensity. The workouts are distributed across the zones according to the level of difficulty. The Green zone is the easiest, progressing to Blue, Purple, Yellow, and Orange with increasing degrees of difficulty. The Red workouts are the most challenging.

The first workout in each zone is the least demanding, and the workouts gradually increase in difficulty up to the last, most demanding session in that zone. The duration of the workouts is determined by how many minutes it takes to complete. Intensity is determined by how hard the workout feels (your perceived exertion).

WORKOUT COLOR ZONES			
Zone (chapter)	Type of workout	RPE	Time
Green (6)	Low intensity, short duration	1-4	≤40 min
Blue (7)	Low intensity, long duration	1-4	≥40 min
Purple (8)	Medium intensity, short duration	5-7	≤50 min
Yellow (9)	Medium intensity, long duration	5-7	≥50 min
Orange (10)	High intensity, short duration	8-10	≤50 min
Red (11)	High intensity, long duration	8-10	≥40 min

Adapted, by permission from T. Iknoian, 1995, *Fitness Walking* (Champaign, IL: Human Kinetics), 50.

Perceived Exertion

Some fitness programs base their measurements of exercise intensity on checking pulse rates, then computing percentages of maximal heart rate to determine how hard you are, or should be, working. Although it is an effective method, it can be cumbersome.

We recommend that you monitor your intensity by judging how easy or hard the workout feels. Your effort should be your intensity guide throughout your workouts. This book describes perceived workout efforts as easy, moderate, and challenging, and these categories pair up rather loosely to the beginning, frequent, and advanced aerobics step exerciser.

Perceived exertion ratings are technically computed as percentages of estimated maximal heart rates. Asking yourself, "How do I feel?" is the quickest, easiest way to tell if you're working too hard, or not hard enough. Many fitness programs are based on this premise. For example, during your workout are you breathless and unable to speak, or is the workout so easy that you could sing two verses of "Star Spangled Banner"? A breathless response should tell you that your exertion is extremely high and you should slow down.

Dr. Gunnar Borg originally devised a 20-point scale of rating perceived exertion to identify levels of intensity, which he later converted to a 10-point rating scale with the help of Dr. Bruce Noble. He found that an individual's sense of how difficult exercise feels correlates very closely with objective measurements of exertion such as maximal oxygen uptake ($\dot{V}O_2$max) and percent of estimated maximal heart rates. We've revised the Borg-Noble scale to coordinate with low, medium, and high intensity efforts.

As you can see from the Workout Color Zones chart, the Green and Blue workouts correlate to an RPE (rating of perceived exertion) score of 1 to 4. Purple and Yellow workouts score 5 to 7, and Orange and Red workouts score 8 to 10.

Caloric Cost

Stepping is a great way to burn energy. Most weight-conscious individuals pay attention to how many kilocalories they burn during activity. The following table gives estimates of your calorie expenditure based on the color-coded workout zones.

Although it is difficult to be precise, we are able to give fairly accurate, conservative estimates. The calculations are based on an average 125-pound stepper. Add 10 percent to these totals for each 15 pounds over 125, and subtract 10 percent for each 15 pounds under 125.

A 125-pound person who engages in a Blue step workout for 40 minutes using a 4-inch step would burn approximately 240 calories (kcal):

$$6 \text{ calories per minute} \times 40 \text{ minutes} = 240 \text{ kcal}$$

A 140-pound individual who does the same workout would burn approximately 264 calories.

$$240 \text{ kcal} + (.10 \times 240 \text{ kcal}) = 264 \text{ kcal}$$

Table II.1
Estimated Caloric Costs of Stepping

Zone	Step height	Kcal/minute	Workout	Total kcals*
Green	4 in.	6	<30 min	≤180
Blue	4 in.	6	>30 min	>180
Purple	8 in.	8	<30 min	≤240
Yellow	8 in.	8	>30 min	>240
Orange	10 in.†	9	<30 min	≤270
Red	10 in.†	9	>30 min	>270

Note. The calculated calorie expenditures are appromiations and do not include those calories burned during warm-up or cool-down phases of the workouts. All calorie calculations are based on a stepping speed of 120 steps per minute (30 step cycles per minute).

*Doing the recommended warm-up, cool-down, and strengthening activities as well as raising workout intensities will increase the amount of kcals burned in all the zones.

†Individuals with orthopedic concerns may choose to continue stepping on an 8-inch step in these zones, because the increase in step height may increase the risk of aggravating joint conditions.

6

Green Zone

The Green zone workouts are the easiest of all the zones. They are low in intensity and fairly short in duration. They carry a rating of perceived exertion (RPE) of between 1 and 4, and they last 30 minutes or less. These workouts should be done by beginners, but they can also be done by experienced steppers who want to ease off from their normal intensity or who have time for only a quick workout. The calorie expenditures for each workout are calculated based on a 4-inch step. Using a higher step will burn more calories per workout.

The 10 Green workout routines are adaptable to all levels of exercisers and incorporate four basic routines.

- **Combo step.** This is the beginning step workout. You'll simply combine movements on and off the step to acclimate your body to this new workout regimen.
- **Steady step.** In this workout, you'll maintain a steady, fluid, uninterrupted pace.
- **Circuit step.** You'll be changing your activity every three minutes in this workout program. The intensity will remain consistently low.
- **Easy interval step.** Interval workouts alternate short, higher intensity step moves with longer, easier recovery moves. Intervals allow you to do more work than you could do continuously.

COMBO STEP

TOTAL TIME: 20-25 minutes

WARM-UP: March in place, tap the top of your step with alternating feet, and march atop the step for 5 minutes.
BEATS PER MINUTE: 118-120
TIME: 10-15 minutes

MOVEMENTS

Alternate lead legs every 1-2 minutes.

Starting position: Front
  Single lead basic step
  Single lead V step
  Marching on the floor.

EFFORT: RPE 2-4
COOL-DOWN: March in place and tap the top of the step with alternating feet for 3-5 minutes.
APPROXIMATE CALORIES BURNED: 60-90

COMMENTS

Remember to alternate lead legs every few minutes. March in place between stepping movements to keep moving for the entire duration of the workout. For example, do a right leg lead basic step for 1 minute, march on the floor for 1 minute, do a left leg lead basic step for 1 minute, then march on floor for 1 minute.

COMBO STEP

TOTAL TIME: 30-35 minutes

WARM-UP: March in place, tap the top of your step with alternating feet, and march atop the step for 5 minutes.
BEATS PER MINUTE: 120
TIME: 15-20 minutes

MOVEMENTS

Starting position: Front
  Single lead basic step
  Single lead V step
  Single lead tap up
  March on the floor.
  Walk around your step.

EFFORT: RPE 2-4
COOL-DOWN: Tap your step with alternating feet, march on the floor, and do easy lunging from side to side for 3-5 minutes. When lunging, make sure your knee remains aligned over your heel, not over your toe. You may need to widen your stance to keep this alignment. Strengthening and stretching exercises for 3-5 minutes.
APPROXIMATE CALORIES BURNED: 120-150

COMMENTS

As you alternate lead legs every 1 minute, try adding the floor movements (marching in place, walking around your step) after 2 or more minutes of continuous stepping. The objective is to try to accomplish nonstop stepping for a longer time than in workout 1.

For example:

Part 1 Sequence

Right leg lead basic step
Left leg lead basic step
March on the floor
Repeat the sequence.

Part 2 Sequence

Right foot lead tap up
Left foot lead tap up
March on the floor
Repeat the sequence.

Part 3 Sequence

Right foot lead over the top
March on the floor

Now, repeat the sequence with the opposite lead leg.

COMBO STEP

TOTAL TIME: 35-45 minutes

WARM-UP: March in place, tap the top of your step with alternating feet, and march atop the step for 5 minutes.
BEATS PER MINUTE: 120
TIME: 20-25 minutes

MOVEMENTS

Starting position: Front
Single lead basic step
Single lead V step
Single lead knee up
Turn step
Over the top
March on the floor.
Walk around your step.
Repeat with opposite lead leg.

EFFORT: RPE 2-4
COOL-DOWN: Tap your step with alternating feet, march on the floor, and do easy lunging from side to side for 3-5 minutes. Strengthening and stretching exercises for 3-5 minutes.
APPROXIMATE CALORIES BURNED: 210-270

COMMENTS

Alternate lead legs every 1 minute. Try adding the floor movements after 5 or more minutes of continuous stepping as well as adding some arm movements (curl ups, upright rows, press downs). The objective is to try to accomplish nonstop stepping for a longer time than in workout 2.

STEADY STEP

TOTAL TIME: 25-30 minutes

WARM-UP: March in place, tap the top of your step with alternating feet, march atop the step, and do alternating basic steps at half-time speed for 5 minutes.
BEATS PER MINUTE: 120
TIME: 10-15 minutes

MOVEMENTS

Starting position: Front
  Right foot basic step with curl ups
  Left foot basic step with curl ups
  Left foot V step with upright rows
  Right foot V step with upright rows
  Right foot tap up with press downs
  Left foot tap up with press downs
  Repeat.

EFFORT: RPE 2-4
COOL-DOWN: Tap your step with alternating feet, march on the floor, and do easy lunging from side to side for 3-5 minutes. Strengthening and stretching exercises for 3-5 minutes.
APPROXIMATE CALORIES BURNED: 60-90

COMMENTS

Spend 1 minute doing each movement. To make lead leg changes, tap the nonoriginating lead foot on the floor. As you become more experienced with the movements, reduce the amount of time for each movement. Try to avoid any walking on the floor. Half-time speed refers to significantly slowing the movement. For example, with a basic step, instead of stepping up with the right foot on count 1, up with the left foot on 2, down with the right foot on 3, followed by the left foot on 4, you would step up with the right foot on counts 1 and 2, up with the left foot on counts 3 and 4, down with the right foot on counts 5 and 6, and down with the left foot on counts 7 and 8.

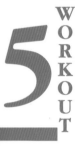

STEADY STEP

5

TOTAL TIME: 30-40 minutes

WARM-UP: March in place, tap the top of the step with alternating feet, march atop the step, and do alternating basic steps at half-time speed for 5 minutes. Incorporate free-flowing arm movements into the warm-up (arm circles, shoulder shrugs, overhead reaches).
BEATS PER MINUTE: 120
TIME: 15-20 minutes

MOVEMENTS

Starting position: Top (heels near the short end)
Straddle down with right leg leading with press downs
Basic step down with right leg leading with free-arm swings
Tap down with right leg leading with press downs
8 lunges with right leg leading with upright rows
Repeat sequence with left leg leading.

EFFORT: RPE 3-4
COOL-DOWN: Tap your step with alternating feet, march on the floor, and do easy lunging from side to side for 3-5 minutes. Strengthening and stretching exercises for 3-5 minutes.
APPROXIMATE CALORIES BURNED: 180-240

COMMENTS

Spend 1 minute doing each movement. To make lead leg changes, tap the nonoriginating lead foot on the top of the step. As you become more experienced with the movements, reduce the amount of time for each movement. Keep moving for the entire workout. If you become excessively fatigued, go back to the previous workout.

STEADY STEP

TOTAL TIME: 40-50 minutes

WARM-UP: March in place, tap the top of your step with alternating feet, march atop the step, and do alternating basic steps at half-time speed for 5 minutes. Incorporate free-flowing arm movements into the warm-up (arm circles, shoulder shrugs, overhead reaches).
BEATS PER MINUTE: 120
TIME: 25-30 minutes

MOVEMENTS

(Putting together two sequences with different starting positions)

Starting position: Front
  Right foot basic step with curl ups
  Left foot basic step with curl ups
  Left foot V step with upright rows
  Right foot V step with upright rows
  Right foot tap up with press downs
  Left foot tap up with press downs
  Repeat.

Starting position: Top (heels near the short end)
  Straddle down with right leg leading with press downs
  Basic step down with right leg leading with free-arm swings
  Tap down with right leg leading with press downs
  8 lunges with right leg leading with upright rows
  Repeat sequence with left leg leading.

EFFORT: RPE 3-4
COOL-DOWN: Tap your step with alternating feet, march on the floor, and do easy lunging from side to side for 3-5 minutes. Strengthening and stretching exercises for 3-5 minutes.
APPROXIMATE CALORIES BURNED: 72-120

COMMENTS

To get from the front position to the top position after you've completed the last segment of the front position combination, stand atop your step heels near the short end. Wait for the musical downbeat, then begin the second combination. Continue alternating the two combinations for the duration of the workout.

STEADY STEP

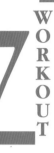

W O R K O U T

7

TOTAL TIME: 40-50 minutes

WARM-UP: March in place, tap the top of your step with alternating feet, march atop the step, and do alternating basic steps at half-time speed for 5 minutes. Incorporate free-flowing arm movements into the warm-up (arm circles, shoulder shrugs, overhead reaches).
BEATS PER MINUTE: 120
TIME: 25-30 minutes

MOVEMENTS

(Putting together three sequences)
Starting position: Front
  Single lead basic step
  Single lead V step
  Single lead knee up
  Turn step
  Over the top
  Repeat with the opposite lead leg.

Starting position: Front
  Right foot basic step with curl ups
  Left foot basic step with curl ups
  Left foot V step with upright rows
  Right foot V step with upright rows
  Right foot tap up with press downs

Left foot tap up with press downs
Repeat.

Starting position: Top (heels near the short end)
  Straddle down with right leg leading with press downs
  Basic step down with right leg leading with free-arm swings
  Tap down with right leg leading with press downs
  8 lunges with right leg leading with upright rows
  Repeat 3rd sequence with left leg leading.

EFFORT: RPE 3-4
COOL-DOWN: Tap your step with alternating feet, march on the floor, and do easy lunging from side to side for 3-5 minutes. Strengthening and stretching exercises for 3-5 minutes.
APPROXIMATE CALORIES BURNED: 150-180

COMMENTS

This workout is reserved for steppers who can complete workouts 1 through 6 with ease.

CIRCUIT STEP

TOTAL TIME: 25-30 minutes

WARM-UP: March in place, tap the top of your step with alternating feet, march atop the step, and do alternating basic steps at half-time speed for 5 minutes. Incorporate free-flowing arm movements into the warm-up (arm circles, shoulder shrugs, overhead reaches). ·
BEATS PER MINUTE: 120
TIME: 12-16 minutes

MOVEMENTS

Alternate 3 minutes of step with 1 minute of strengthening exercises for a great total-body step workout.

Starting position: Side

Over the top with pull back arms	3 minutes
Squats with one foot atop the step	1 minute
Over the top with pull back arms	3 minutes
Squat with opposite foot atop the step	1 minute

Starting position: Front

Alternating knee up with free-style arms	3 minutes
Alternating single leg lunge with curl ups	1 minute
Turn step with press downs	3 minutes
Alternating single leg lunge with arm reaches	1 minute

EFFORT: RPE 3-4
COOL-DOWN: Tap your step with alternating feet, march on the floor, and do easy lunging from side to side for 3-5 minutes, then stretch for 3-5 minutes.
APPROXIMATE CALORIES BURNED: 72-90

COMMENTS

This workout provides you with an alternative to your steady step workout. It strengthens your muscles. You don't need to do additional lower body strengthening exercises with this workout. You may want to do a set of abdominal and back exercises, though.

EASY INTERVAL STEP

TOTAL TIME: 25-30 minutes

WARM-UP: March in place, tap the top of your step with alternating feet, march atop the step, and do alternating basic steps at half-time speed for 5 minutes. Incorporate free-flowing arm movements into the warm-up (arm circles, shoulder shrugs, overhead reaches).

BEATS PER MINUTE: 120

TIME: 16 minutes

MOVEMENTS

Alternate 3 minutes of easy step moves with 1 minute of high intensity step moves.

Starting position: Top (facing the short end of the step)

Alternating lead straddle down with press downs	3 minutes
Alternating lunge with arm reaches	1 minute
Alternating basic step down with pull backs	3 minutes
Alternating lunge with arm reaches	1 minute

Repeat for the remainder of the workout.

EFFORT: Average RPE 4 (2-6 range)

COOL-DOWN: Tap your step with alternating feet, march on the floor, and do easy lunging from side to side for 3-5 minutes. Strengthening and stretching exercises for 3-5 minutes.

APPROXIMATE CALORIES BURNED: 96

COMMENTS

This workout provides you with a challenging alternative to your step program. It allows for maximum calorie expenditure in a short amount of time. During the 1-minute intervals, your breathing rate and pulse will increase significantly. Stop if you feel any discomfort. Attempt this workout only if you have successfully completed workouts 1 through 8 in this zone.

EASY INTERVAL STEP

TOTAL TIME: 40-45 minutes

WARM-UP: March in place, tap the top of your step with alternating feet, march atop the step, and do alternating basic steps at half-time speed for 5 minutes. Incorporate free-flowing arm movements into the warm-up (arm circles, shoulder shrugs, overhead reaches).
BEATS PER MINUTE: 120
TIME: 20-30 minutes

MOVEMENTS

Alternate 3 minutes of easy step moves with 1 minute of high intensity step moves.

Starting position: Front

Alternating V step with arm reaches	3 minutes
Alternating repeater with curl ups	1 minute
Alternating basic step with pull backs	3 minutes
Alternating repeater with press downs	1 minute
Turn step with pull backs	3 minutes
Alternating power leap up	1 minute

Repeat for the remainder of the workout.

EFFORT: Average RPE 4 (2-6 range)
COOL-DOWN: Tap your step with alternating feet, march on the floor, and do easy lunging from side to side for 3-5 minutes. Strengthening and stretching exercises for 3-5 minutes.
APPROXIMATE CALORIES BURNED: 120-180

COMMENTS

Save this workout for those days you feel like having a challenge!

	Green Zone Summary		
Workout	Description	Total duration (minutes)	Intensity (RPE)
1	Combo step	20-25	2-4
2	Combo step	30-35	2-4
3	Combo step	35-45	2-4
4	Steady step	25-30	2-4
5	Steady step	30-40	3-4
6	Steady step	40-50	3-4
7	Steady step	40-50	3-4
8	Circuit step	25-30	3-4
9	Easy interval step	25-30	4
10	Easy interval step	40-45	4

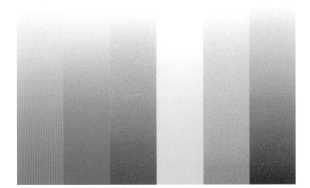

7

Blue Zone

Blue zone workouts are similar in content, effort, and execution to the workouts in the Green zone. Blue zone workouts score a rating between 1 and 4 on perceived exertion and offer the same benefits as the Green zone workouts. The calorie expenditures are still calculated based on a four-inch step. The major difference between the Green and Blue workouts is the duration. Blue zone workouts last longer. Thirty minutes will now become the lower instead of the upper boundary.

The 10 Blue workouts are attainable by most step exercisers. Your current training level will help determine if the longest workouts in this chapter are within your grasp. The longest workout in this chapter allows you the opportunity to exercise at a comfortable pace for an extended amount of time. It lets your mind and spirit drift as you stay motivated by your music and the fun movements you're performing.

COMBO STEP

1 WORKOUT

TOTAL TIME: 40-50 minutes

WARM-UP: Slow stepping alternated with walking on the floor for 5 minutes
BEATS PER MINUTE: 118-120
TIME: 30-40 minutes

MOVEMENTS

Alternate lead legs every 1-2 minutes.

Starting position: Front
  Single lead basic step
  Single lead V step
  Single lead tap up
  March on the floor.

EFFORT: RPE 2-4
COOL-DOWN: March in place and tap the top of the step with alternating feet for 3-5 minutes. Strengthening and stretching exercises for 3-5 minutes.
APPROXIMATE CALORIES BURNED: 180-240

COMMENTS

Alternate step movements with marching on the floor every 2-3 minutes. Be creative with your floor movements. Try marching with style, high knees, cha-chas, and other fun variations. A cha-cha is a triple step (counted 1 & 2), and is also known as a "polka step."

COMBO STEP

TOTAL TIME: 45-60 minutes

WARM-UP: Marching in place, slow stepping, and tapping the top of the step for 5 minutes
BEATS PER MINUTE: 120
TIME: 35-45 minutes

MOVEMENTS

Alternate lead legs every 1-2 minutes.
Starting position: Front
  Single lead basic step
  Single lead V step
  Single lead tap up
  Single lead knee up
  Turn step
  March on the floor.

EFFORT: RPE 2-4
COOL-DOWN: Tap your step with alternating feet, march on the floor, and do easy lunging from side to side for 3-5 minutes. Strengthening and stretching exercises for 3-5 minutes.
APPROXIMATE CALORIES BURNED: 210-300

COMMENTS

Incorporate floor moves every 2-3 minutes. Your effort should remain low throughout this workout. You should not be breathless or excessively fatigued.

COMBO STEP

TOTAL TIME: 50-65 minutes

WARM-UP: March in place, tap the top of your step with alternating feet, and do a slow step for 5 minutes.
BEATS PER MINUTE: 120
TIME: 40-50 minutes

MOVEMENTS

Alternate lead legs after 1 minute of stepping.

Starting position: Front
  Single lead basic step
  Single lead V step
  Single lead knee up
  Turn step
  Over the top
  March on the floor.
  Repeat from beginning with the opposite lead leg.

EFFORT: RPE 2-4
COOL-DOWN: Tap your step with alternating feet, march on the floor, and do lunges from side to side for 3-5 minutes. Strengthening and stretching exercises for 3-5 minutes.
APPROXIMATE CALORIES BURNED: 240-360

COMMENTS

Try stepping for extended periods (that is, 3 to 4 movements) before integrating floor moves. Try adding upper body movements as you step (curl ups, press downs, arm reaches).

STEADY STEP

TOTAL TIME: 40-50 minutes

WARM-UP: March in place, tap the top of your step with alternating feet, and do slow stepping for 5 minutes.
BEATS PER MINUTE: 120
TIME: 30-35 minutes

MOVEMENTS

Starting position: Front
  Right foot basic step with curl ups
  Left foot basic step with curl ups
  Left foot V step with upright rows
  Right foot V step with upright rows
  Right foot tap up with press downs
  Left foot tap up with press downs
  Repeat for remainder of workout.

EFFORT: RPE 2-4
COOL-DOWN: Tap your step with alternating feet, march on the floor, and lunge from side to side for 3-5 minutes. Strengthening and stretching exercises for 3-5 minutes.
APPROXIMATE CALORIES BURNED: 180-240

COMMENTS

Spend 1-2 minutes doing each movement. Take your time with this workout. Avoid incorporating any floor movements. If this workout seems unusually challenging, go back to workout 3.

STEADY STEP

W O R K O U T

TOTAL TIME: 45-60 minutes

WARM-UP: March in place, tap the top of your step, and do slow stepping for 5 minutes.
BEATS PER MINUTE: 120
TIME: 35-45 minutes

MOVEMENTS

Starting position: Top (heels near the short end)
  Straddle down with right leg leading with press downs
  Basic step down with right leg leading with free-arm swings
  Tap down with right leg leading with press downs
  8 lunges with right leg leading with upright rows
  Repeat the sequence with left leg leading.

EFFORT: RPE 3-4
COOL-DOWN: Tap your step with alternating feet, march on the floor, and do lunges side to side for 3-5 minutes. Strengthening and stretching exercises for 3-5 minutes.
APPROXIMATE CALORIES BURNED: 210-300

COMMENTS

Remember to change lead legs for each movement after approximately 1 minute. Keep moving for the entire time suggested. Pace yourself, and enjoy!

STEADY STEP

TOTAL TIME: 60-75 minutes

WARM-UP: March in place, tap the top of your step with alternating feet, march atop the step, and do slow stepping with free-flowing arm movements for 5 minutes.
BEATS PER MINUTE: 120
TIME: 50-60 minutes

MOVEMENTS

(Putting together two sequences with varying starting positions)

Starting position: Front
  Right foot basic step with curl ups
  Left foot basic step with curl ups
  Left foot V step with upright rows
  Right foot V step with upright rows
  Right foot tap up with press downs
  Left foot tap up with press downs
  Repeat.

Starting position: Top (facing the short end)
  Right leg straddle down with press downs
  Right leg basic step down with free-swinging arms
  Right leg tap down with press downs
  Right leg lunge for eight repetitions with upright rows
  Repeat 2nd sequence with left leg leading.

EFFORT: RPE 3-4
COOL-DOWN: Tap step with alternating feet, march on the floor, and lunge from side to side for 3-5 minutes. Strengthening and stretching exercises for 3-5 minutes.
APPROXIMATE CALORIES BURNED: 300-360

COMMENTS

To avoid boredom, feel free to change arm movements or add other starting positions to the movements. Try alternating leads after every 8 counts for variety. If you think you'll have trouble stepping for this length of time, do some walking on the floor for breaks.

STEADY STEP

WORKOUT 7

TOTAL TIME: 65-80 minutes

WARM-UP: March in place, tap your step, and do slow stepping for 5 minutes. Add arm movements of your choice.
BEATS PER MINUTE: 120
TIME: 55-65 minutes

MOVEMENTS

(Putting together three sequences)

Starting position: Front
Single lead basic step
Single lead V step
Single lead knee up
Turn step
Over the top
Repeat with opposite lead leg.

Starting position: Front
Right foot basic step with curl ups
Left foot basic step with curl ups
Left foot V step with upright rows
Right foot V step with upright rows
Right foot tap up with press downs
Left foot tap up with press downs
Repeat.

Starting position: Top (heels near the short end)
Right leg straddle down with press downs
Right leg basic step down with free-swinging arms
Right leg tap down with press downs
Right leg lunge for eight repetitions with upright rows
Repeat 3rd sequence with left leg leading.

EFFORT: RPE 3-4
COOL-DOWN: Tap your step with alternating feet, march on the floor, and lunge from side to side for 3-5 minutes. Strengthening and stretching exercises for 3-5 minutes.
APPROXIMATE CALORIES BURNED: 330-450

COMMENTS

Schedule this workout on a day when you have the most free time. Pay attention to signs of overuse injuries, such as sore knees, back, and ankles.

CIRCUIT STEP

TOTAL TIME: 60-75 minutes

WARM-UP: March in place, tap the top of your step, and do slow stepping for 5 minutes. Incorporate arm movements at your leisure.
BEATS PER MINUTE: 120
TIME: 50-60 minutes

MOVEMENTS

Alternate 3 minutes of step with 1 minute of strengthening exercises for a total-body step workout.

Starting position: Side

Over the top with pull backs	3 minutes
Squat with one foot atop the step	1 minute
Over the top with pull downs	3 minutes
Squat with opposite foot atop the step	1 minute
Turn step	3 minutes
Squat with one foot atop the step	1 minute
Alternating knee up	3 minutes
Squat with opposite foot atop the step	1 minute
Repeat.	

EFFORT: RPE 3-4
COOL-DOWN: Tap your step with alternating feet, march on the floor, and lunge from side to side for 3-5 minutes. Abdominal and back strengthening exercises for 3-5 minutes.
APPROXIMATE CALORIES BURNED: 300-390

COMMENTS

Remember to keep the weight over your heels during the squats. If squats become uncomfortable, substitute other standing strengthening exercises, like lunges.

EASY INTERVAL STEP

W
O
R
K
O
U
T

9

TOTAL TIME: 45-60 minutes

WARM-UP: March in place, tap the top of your step with alternating feet, slow step, and march atop the step for 5 minutes. Add upper body movements.
BEATS PER MINUTE: 120
TIME: 35-45 minutes

MOVEMENTS

Alternate 3 minutes of easy step moves with 1 minute of high intensity step moves.

Starting position: Top (heels near the short end)

Alternating straddle down with press downs	3 minutes
Alternating lunge with arm reaches	1 minute
Alternating basic step down with pull backs	3 minutes
Alternating lunge with arm reaches	1 minute

Starting position: Side

Over the top with arm reaches	3 minutes
Turn step with curl ups	1 minute

Repeat for the remainder of the workout.

EFFORT: Average RPE 4 (2-6 range)
COOL-DOWN: Tap your step with alternating feet, march on the floor, and lunge from side to side for 3-5 minutes. Strengthening and stretching exercises for 3-5 minutes.
APPROXIMATE CALORIES BURNED: 210-240

COMMENTS

Using a stopwatch helps keep your intervals on track with the designated workout. Pay careful attention to how you're feeling, especially during the high intensity movements.

EASY INTERVAL STEP

TOTAL TIME: 55-75 minutes

WARM-UP: March in place, tap the top of the step with alternating feet, march atop the step, and do slow stepping for 5 minutes. Incorporate arm movements.
BEATS PER MINUTE: 120
TIME: 45-60 minutes

MOVEMENTS

Alternate 3 minutes of easy step moves with 1 minute of high intensity step moves.

Starting position: Front

Alternating V step with arm reaches	3 minutes
Alternating repeater with curl ups	1 minute
Alternating basic step with pull backs	3 minutes
Alternating repeater with press downs	1 minute
Turn step with pull backs	3 minutes
Alternating power leap up	1 minute

Repeat for the remainder of the workout.

EFFORT: Average RPE 4 (2-6 range)
COOL-DOWN: Tap your step with alternating feet, march on the floor, and lunge from side to side for 3-5 minutes. Strengthening and stretching exercises for 3-5 minutes.
APPROXIMATE CALORIES BURNED: 270-360

COMMENTS

Make sure your music is motivating. This workout is a real challenge. Good luck!

Blue Zone Summary			
Workout	**Description**	**Total duration (minutes)**	**Intensity (RPE)**
1	Combo step	40-50	2-4
2	Combo step	45-60	2-4
3	Combo step	50-65	2-4
4	Steady step	40-50	2-4
5	Steady step	45-60	3-4
6	Steady step	60-75	3-4
7	Steady step	65-80	3-4
8	Circuit step	60-75	3-4
9	Easy interval step	45-60	4
10	Easy interval step	55-75	4

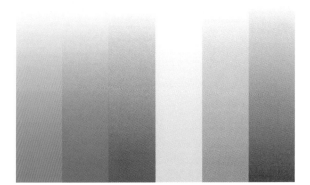

8

Purple Zone

Purple zone workouts are a bit more challenging than the Green and Blue zones. The intensity has been increased, resulting in a rating of perceived exertion in the 5 to 7 range, but the duration is short. All workouts typically include powerful movements. The calorie expenditures are calculated based on an individual's using an 8-inch step. Using a lower step may cause you to burn fewer calories, and using a higher step height may cause you to burn more.

The 10 Purple workouts have been designed with greater variety in the routines. Some routines include steady stepping with moderately challenging movements. Others use interval workouts with very challenging power moves for brief periods, interspersed with recovery periods of lower intensity movements.

Interval workouts are used frequently by athletes to improve their fitness levels. Intervals cause them to train harder for brief periods, which pushes their bodies beyond the levels reached in a steady workout.

Pure, high intensity interval training is not recommended for novice step exercisers because it can increase the risk of injury and fatigue. All interval workouts will alternate 3 minutes of low intensity recovery movements with 1 minute of higher intensity power step movements. During the 1-minute routines, your RPE should reach near 7, in comparison to an RPE of 5 for the 3-minute routines.

COMBO STEP INTERVAL

1 WORKOUT

TOTAL TIME: 30-40 minutes

WARM-UP: March atop the step, march around the step, tap the top of the step with alternating feet, and swing your arms freely for 5 minutes.
BEATS PER MINUTE: 120-126
TIME: 20-25 minutes

MOVEMENTS

Three minutes alternating the following moves:

Starting position: Side
  March in place with arm reaches.
  March around your step with pull backs.
  Step touches
  Repeat, marching around your step in the other direction.

One minute of the following moves:

Starting position: Astride
  Power jump up with arm reaches

Repeat the 3-minute/1-minute interval sequences for the duration of the workout.

EFFORT: RPE 5-7
COOL-DOWN: March in place, around your step, and atop your step. Tap the top of your step with alternating feet for 3-5 minutes. Strengthening and stretching exercises for 3-5 minutes.
APPROXIMATE CALORIES BURNED: 160-200

COMMENTS

You may want to execute all low impact moves on the floor during the 3-minute interval. To increase the intensity of low impact moves, raise your knees higher during the march, and take big side steps during the step touches. The suggested beats per minute have been increased for this workout. If you feel it's too fast, you may select music closer to 120 than to 126 BPM.

COMBO STEP INTERVAL

TOTAL TIME: 35-45 minutes

WARM-UP: March atop the step, march around the step, tap the top of the step with alternating feet, and swing your arms freely for 5 minutes.
BEATS PER MINUTE: 120-126
TIME: 25-30 minutes

MOVEMENTS

Three minutes alternating the following moves:

Starting position: End
  Tap alternating feet atop the step with arm reaches.
  March around your step with press downs.
  Knee up

One minute of the following move:

Starting position: End
  Alternating repeater knee up with arm reaches

Repeat the 3-minute/1-minute interval sequences for the duration of the workout.

EFFORT: RPE 5-7
COOL-DOWN: March in place, around your step, and atop your step. Tap the top of your step with alternating feet for 3-5 minutes. Strengthening and stretching exercises for 3-5 minutes.
APPROXIMATE CALORIES BURNED: 200-280

COMMENTS

To increase the intensity of the knee ups, add a hop and raise your arms overhead, as if you were shooting a basketball.

COMBO STEP INTERVAL

W O R K O U T

3

TOTAL TIME: 45-55 minutes

WARM-UP: Slow stepping alternated with walking on the floor for 5 minutes
BEATS PER MINUTE: 120-126
TIME: 35-40 minutes

MOVEMENTS

Three minutes alternating the following moves:

Starting position: Front
  March in place with fun-time arms.
  Alternating knee up
  Step touch or jumping jack
  Tap alternating heels atop the step.

One minute of the following move:

Starting position: Top
  Alternating lunge with fun-time arms

Repeat the 3-minute/1-minute routines for the remainder of the workout.

EFFORT: RPE 5-7
COOL-DOWN: March in place, around your step, and atop your step. Tap the top of your step with alternating feet for 3-5 minutes. Strengthening and stretching exercises for 3-5 minutes.
APPROXIMATE CALORIES BURNED: 280-360

COMMENTS

Remember to keep an upright torso during the lunges. Touch only the ball of the foot on the floor while your knee and hip remain aligned over, not in front of, your ankle region.

TONING STEP INTERVAL

TOTAL TIME: 30-40 minutes

WARM-UP: Slow stepping alternated, marching in place on the floor and atop the step, followed by stationary half squats for 5 minutes
BEATS PER MINUTE: 120-126
TIME: 20-25 minutes

MOVEMENTS

Three minutes alternating the following moves:

Starting position: Top
  Single leg stationary lunge with right foot atop the step
  Single leg stationary lunge with left foot atop the step

One minute of the following move:

Starting position: Front
  Alternating power leap up with fun-time arms

Repeat the 3-minute/1-minute routines for the remainder of the workout.

EFFORT: RPE 5-7
COOL-DOWN: March in place, around your step, and atop your step. Tap the top of your step with alternating feet for 3-5 minutes. Abdominal and back strengthening exercises for 3-5 minutes (optional, because the 3-minute interval focuses on strength exercises), then stretch.
APPROXIMATE CALORIES BURNED: 160-200

COMMENTS

If you have knee problems, you can do half lunges and squats. Don't work to the point of pain. All exercises should be somewhat challenging but still comfortable. When lunging and squatting, remember to keep your neutral posture: hips above knee level, and knees, hips, and ankles aligned.

TONING STEP INTERVAL

5 WORKOUT

TOTAL TIME: 35-45 minutes

WARM-UP: Slow stepping alternated, marching in place on the floor and atop the step, followed by stationary half squats for 5 minutes
BEATS PER MINUTE: 120-126
TIME: 25-30 minutes

MOVEMENTS

Three minutes alternating the following moves:

Starting position: Front
 Single leg stationary lunge with right foot atop the step
 Single leg stationary lunge with left foot atop the step

Starting position: Side
 Squat with right foot atop the step
 Squat with left foot atop the step

One minute of the following move:

Starting position: Front
 Alternating repeater with arm reaches

Repeat the 3-minute/1-minute routines for the remainder of the workout.

EFFORT: RPE 5-7
COOL-DOWN: March in place, around your step, and atop your step. Tap the top of your step with alternating feet for 3-5 minutes. Abdominal and back strengthening exercises for 3-5 minutes (optional, because the 3-minute interval focuses on strength exercises), then stretch.
APPROXIMATE CALORIES BURNED: 200-280

COMMENTS

To vary the squat exercise, keep your heel lifted, which increases work of the gastrocnemius (calf) muscle.

TONING STEP INTERVAL

TOTAL TIME: 45-55 minutes

WARM-UP: Slow stepping alternated, marching in place on the floor and atop the step, followed by stationary half squats for 5 minutes
BEATS PER MINUTE: 120-126
TIME: 35-40 minutes

MOVEMENTS

Three minutes alternating the following moves:

Starting position: Front
  Single leg stationary lunge with right foot atop the step
  Single leg stationary lunge with left foot atop the step

Starting position: Side
  Squat with right foot atop the step
  Squat with left foot atop the step

Starting position: Top
  Alternating slow lunge

One minute of the following move:

Starting position: Astride
  Power jump up with arm reaches

Repeat the 3-minute/1-minute routines for the remainder of the workout.

EFFORT: RPE 5-7
COOL-DOWN: March in place, around your step, and atop your step. Tap the top of your step with alternating feet for 3-5 minutes. Abdominal and back strengthening exercises for 3-5 minutes (optional, because the 3-minute interval focuses on strength exercises), then stretch.
APPROXIMATE CALORIES BURNED: 280-360

COMMENTS

Pay careful attention to your alignment and execution, especially during the lunges.

POWER STEP INTERVAL

WORKOUT 7

TOTAL TIME: 25-35 minutes

WARM-UP: Slow stepping alternated with walking on the floor for 5 minutes

BEATS PER MINUTE: 120-126

TIME: 15-20 minutes

MOVEMENTS

Three minutes alternating the following moves:

Starting position: Front
  Single lead basic step with arm reaches
  Single lead V step with upright rows
  Single lead tap up with arm reaches
  Over the top with press downs
  Repeat with alternate leg leading.

One minute of the following move:

Starting position: Front
  Alternating power leap up with fun-time arms

Repeat the 3-minute/1-minute routines for the remainder of the workout.

EFFORT: RPE 5-7

COOL-DOWN: March in place, around your step, and atop your step. Tap the top of your step with alternating feet for 3-5 minutes. Strengthening and stretching exercises for 3-5 minutes.

APPROXIMATE CALORIES BURNED: 160-200

COMMENTS

If you find it difficult to step at the suggested speed, slow the tempo down or lower your step.

POWER STEP INTERVAL

TOTAL TIME: 35-45 minutes

WARM-UP: Slow stepping alternated with walking on the floor for 5 minutes
BEATS PER MINUTE: 120-126
TIME: 25-30 minutes

MOVEMENTS

Three minutes alternating the following moves:

Starting position: Front
  Single lead basic step with arm reaches
  Single lead V step with upright rows
  Single lead tap up with arm reaches
  Over the top with press downs
  Repeat with alternate leg leading.

One minute of the following move:

Starting position: Top
  Alternating lead lunge with fun-time arms

Repeat the 3-minute/1-minute routines for the remainder of the workout.

EFFORT: RPE 5-7
COOL-DOWN: March in place, around your step, and atop your step. Tap the top of your step with alternating feet for 3-5 minutes. Strengthening and stretching exercises for 3-5 minutes.
APPROXIMATE CALORIES BURNED: 200-280

COMMENTS

Have fun adding your own arm movements.

POWER STEP INTERVAL

9

TOTAL TIME: 45-55 minutes

WARM-UP: March in place, do slow stepping, march atop your step, and tap the top of your step with alternating feet for 5 minutes. Add upper body movements that are rhythmic, fluid, and use a full range of motion.
BEATS PER MINUTE: 120-126
TIME: 35-40 minutes

MOVEMENTS

Three minutes alternating the following movements:

Starting position: Front
  Single lead basic step with curl ups
  Single lead tap up with reaches
  Single lead V step with upright rows
  3 turn steps with reaches
  Repeat with alternate leg leading.

One minute of the following move:

Starting position: Front
  Alternating repeater with curl ups

Repeat the 3-minute/1-minute routines for the duration of the workout.

EFFORT: RPE 5-7
COOL-DOWN: March in place, around your step, and atop your step. Tap the top of your step with alternating feet for 3-5 minutes. Strengthening and stretching exercises for 3-5 minutes.
APPROXIMATE CALORIES BURNED: 280-360

COMMENTS

The 3 turn steps help move you to the opposite lead leg. If the 1-minute routine finds you excessively breathless, omit the arm movements and focus on the legs.

POWER STEP INTERVAL

TOTAL TIME: 50-65 minutes

WARM-UP: March in place, tap the top of your step with alternating feet, and march atop your step for 5 minutes.
BEATS PER MINUTE: 120-126
TIME: 40-50 minutes

MOVEMENTS

Three minutes alternating the following moves:

Starting position: Front
  Alternating lead knee up with reaches
  Alternating lead basic step with fun-time arms
  Turn step
  Alternating lead V step with press downs

One minute of the following move:

Starting position: Astride
  Power jump up

EFFORT: RPE 5-7
COOL-DOWN: March in place, around your step, and atop your step. Tap the top of your step with alternating feet for 3-5 minutes. Strengthening and stretching exercises for 3-5 minutes.
APPROXIMATE CALORIES BURNED: 320-400

COMMENTS

If you're having difficulty with the power jump up, reach your arms upward as you're jumping. The momentum of your arms coupled with the legs will make this move easier.

Purple Zone Summary			
Workout	**Description**	**Total duration (minutes)**	**Intensity (RPE)**
1	Combo step interval	30-40	5-7
2	Combo step interval	35-45	5-7
3	Combo step interval	45-55	5-7
4	Toning step interval	30-40	5-7
5	Toning step interval	35-45	5-7
6	Toning step interval	45-55	5-7
7	Power step interval	25-35	5-7
8	Power step interval	35-45	5-7
9	Power step interval	45-55	5-7
10	Power step interval	50-65	5-7

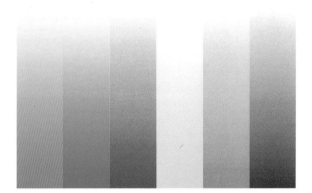

9

Yellow Zone

In the Yellow zone, by increasing the duration, we take your workouts a bit further than those you experienced in the Purple zone. The intensity continues to fall between a perceived exertion rating range of 5 to 7. Yellow workouts are longer, lasting more than 30 minutes each. The calorie expenditures are calculated based on an individual using an 8-inch step. Using a lower step may burn fewer calories, and using a higher step may burn more.

There won't be any new movement elements to your program in this chapter, so you'll have the opportunity to concentrate on your execution while achieving success with each workout. You'll notice some dramatic duration increases, which award extra calorie burning.

The 10 Yellow workouts are best for the intermediate step exerciser desiring a longer workout at an easy to moderate intensity. These workouts are great to do on days when you have a bit more time for exercising.

**W
O
R
K
O
U
T**

1

TOTAL TIME: 50-60 minutes

WARM-UP: Step on the platform, march on the floor, and alternate toe taps atop the platform while swinging your arms freely in the fullest range of motion for 5 minutes.
BEATS PER MINUTE: 120-126
TIME: 40-45 minutes

MOVEMENTS

Three minutes alternating the following moves:

Starting position: Side
  March in place with arm reaches.
  March around your step with pull backs.
  Jumping jack or knee up
  Repeat, marching around your step in the other direction.

One minute alternating the following moves:

Starting position: Astride
  Power jump up with arm reaches
  Alternating straddle up

Repeat the 3-minute/1-minute interval sequences for the duration of the workout.

EFFORT: RPE 5-7
COOL-DOWN: March in place, around your step, and atop your step. Tap the top of your step with alternating feet for 3-5 minutes. Strengthening and stretching exercises for 3-5 minutes.
APPROXIMATE CALORIES BURNED: 280-400

COMMENTS

Remember to maintain an easy intensity throughout this combo step workout. The goal is not to push to the point of exhaustion.

TOTAL TIME: 55-65 minutes

WARM-UP: March atop the step, around the step, and in place. Tap the top of the step with alternating feet. Include free-flowing arm movements that use full range of motion for 5 minutes.
BEATS PER MINUTE: 120-126
TIME: 45-50 minutes

MOVEMENTS

Three minutes alternating the following moves:

Starting position: End
  Tap alternating feet atop the step with arm reaches.
  March around your step with press downs.
  Knee up

One minute alternating the following moves:

Starting position: End
  Alternating repeater with arm reaches
  Alternating basic step with curl ups

EFFORT: RPE 5-7
COOL-DOWN: March in place, around your step, and atop your step. Tap the top of your step with alternating feet for 3-5 minutes. Strengthening and stretching exercises for 3-5 minutes.
APPROXIMATE CALORIES BURNED: 320-440

COMMENTS

Challenge yourself during the 1-minute step segment by changing the basic step to a power-basic step. To execute a power-basic step, leap atop the platform with the right foot followed by the left foot, then step down with the right followed by the left. The cadence is run, run, step down, step down. Don't forget about your posture!

3 WORKOUT

TOTAL TIME: 60-75 minutes

WARM-UP: Slow stepping alternated with walking on the floor incorporating a full range of motion with arm movements for 5 minutes
BEATS PER MINUTE: 120-126
TIME: 55-60 minutes

MOVEMENTS

Three minutes alternating the following moves:

Starting position: Front
   March in place with fun-time arms.
   Alternating knee up with arm reaches
   Step touch or jumping jack
   Tap alternating heels atop the step.

One minute alternating the following moves:

Starting position: Top
   Alternating lunge with curl ups
   Alternating basic step down with pull backs

Repeat the 3-minute/1-minute routines for the remainder of the workout.

EFFORT: RPE 5-7
COOL-DOWN: March in place, around your step, and atop your step. Tap the top of your step with alternating feet for 3-5 minutes. Strengthening and stretching exercises for 3-5 minutes.
APPROXIMATE CALORIES BURNED: 440-480

COMMENTS

As the workout time increases, you may feel the need to incorporate more floor movement breaks. Take these breaks if needed, especially if you experience any discomfort in your knees, ankles, or back.

TOTAL TIME: 65-80 minutes

WARM-UP: Slow stepping alternated with walking on the floor while incorporating full range of motion with arm movements for 5 minutes
BEATS PER MINUTE: 120-126
TIME: 60-65 minutes

MOVEMENTS

(Putting together two sequences with varying starting positions)

Starting position: Front
  Right foot basic step with curl ups
  Left foot basic step with curl ups
  Left foot V step with upright rows
  Right foot V step with upright rows
  Right foot tap up with press downs
  Left foot tap up with press downs
  Repeat.

Starting position: Top (heels near the short end)
  Right straddle down with press downs
  Right leg basic step down with free-swinging arms
  Right leg tap down with press downs
  Right leg lunge for 8 repetitions with upright rows
  Repeat the sequence with left leg leading.

EFFORT: RPE 5-7
COOL-DOWN: March in place, around your step, and atop your step. Tap the top of your step with alternating feet for 3-5 minutes. Strengthening and stretching exercises for 3-5 minutes.
APPROXIMATE CALORIES BURNED: 480-520

COMMENTS

We have not specified how many repetitions of each step to execute per lead leg, so you have the opportunity to design your own workout. We recommend, though, that you don't spend more than 1 minute of continuous stepping per lead leg per movement.

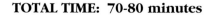

5 WORKOUT

TOTAL TIME: 70-80 minutes

WARM-UP: Slow stepping alternated with walking on the floor while incorporating a full range of motion with arm movements for 5 minutes
BEATS PER MINUTE: 120-126
TIME: 60-65 minutes

MOVEMENTS

Putting together three sequences with varying starting positions

Starting position: Front
  Single lead basic step with arm reaches
  Single lead V step with curl ups
  Single lead knee up with fun-time arms
  Turn step with hand claps
  Repeat with alternate leg leading.

Starting position: Side
  3 tap ups with hand claps
  1 over the top with arm reaches

Starting position: Top (heels near the short end)
  Alternating straddle down with press downs
  Alternating lunge with arm reaches
  Repeat.

EFFORT: RPE 5-7
COOL-DOWN: March in place, around your step, and atop your step. Tap the top of your step with alternating feet for 3-5 minutes. Strengthening and stretching exercises for 3-5 minutes.
APPROXIMATE CALORIES BURNED: 480-560

COMMENTS

Once you're successful at the moves in parts 1 and 2, try mixing and matching them to come up with your own sequence.

LONG STEADY STEP

TOTAL TIME: 70-80 minutes

WARM-UP: Slow stepping alternated with walking on the floor while incorporating a full range of motion with arm movements for 5 minutes
BEATS PER MINUTE: 120-126
TIME: 60-65 minutes

MOVEMENTS

Three sequences with varying starting positions

Starting position: Astride
  Single lead straddle up
  Alternating lead knee up
  Power jump up
  Repeat with opposite leg leading.

Starting position: Top (heels near short end of step)
  Alternating lunge
  Alternating basic step down (Tap foot atop step to change lead legs.)

Starting position: Top (heels near short end of step)
  3 tap downs, right leg lead to the right side
  1 straddle down
  3 tap downs, left leg lead to the left side
  1 straddle down

EFFORT: RPE 5-7
COOL-DOWN: March in place, around your step, and atop your step. Tap the top of your step with alternating feet for 3-5 minutes. Strengthening and stretching exercises for 3-5 minutes.
APPROXIMATE CALORIES BURNED: 520-600

COMMENTS

This routine requires memory skills in addition to movement skills. Challenge yourself by attempting to put 1, 2, or all 3 parts together. Feel free to mix and match the parts you enjoy most.

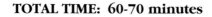

WORKOUT 7

TOTAL TIME: 60-70 minutes

WARM-UP: Slow stepping alternated with walking on the floor while incorporating a full range of motion with arm movements for 5 minutes
BEATS PER MINUTE: 120-126
TIME: 50-55 minutes

MOVEMENTS

Alternate each of the following components for 3 minutes throughout the entire workout.

Component 1
Starting position: Front
  Alternating basic step with curl ups
  Alternating V step with arm reaches
  Alternating knee up with fun-time arms

Component 2
Starting position: Top
  Alternating leg lunge
  Stationary leg lunge with right foot
  Stationary leg lunge with left foot
  Repeat.

Component 3
Starting position: Side
  3 tap ups with press downs
  1 over the top with arm reaches
  4 turn steps with fun-time arms
  Repeat.

Component 4
Starting position: Front
  8 squats with 1 foot atop the step (to the beat of the music)
  March to the other side of the step.
  8 squats with the opposite foot atop the step (to the beat of the music)

EFFORT: RPE 5-7
COOL-DOWN: March in place, around your step, and atop your step. Tap the top of your step with alternating feet for 3-5 minutes. Abdominal and back strengthening exercises for 3-5 minutes (optional), then stretch.
APPROXIMATE CALORIES BURNED: 400-440

COMMENTS

This workout provides a well-rounded program because it combines toning or strengthening exercises with stepping. Try variations of the knee up to add greater variety to the workout. Instead of lifting the knee, try kicking the foot, curling the foot behind while bending the knee, or lifting the leg to the side.

WORKOUT 8

TOTAL TIME: 65-80 minutes

WARM-UP: Slow stepping alternated with walking on the floor while incorporating a full range of motion with arm movements for 5 minutes
BEATS PER MINUTE: 120-126
TIME: 60-65 minutes

MOVEMENTS

Alternate each component for 3 minutes and add your own arm movements throughout the entire workout.

Component 1
Starting position: End
  Alternating basic step
  Alternating knee up with
    variations
  Turn step
  Repeat.

Component 2
Starting position: Top (heels at
the short end of the step)
  Alternating lunge off the step
    (leg going behind)
  Heel raise atop the step

  Alternating slow squat off the
    step (leg going to the side)
  Repeat.

Component 3
Starting position: Side
  Alternating lead over the top
    with arm reaches
  Single lead tap up with press
    downs
  Single lead power leap up
    with fun-time arms
  Repeat with opposite lead legs.
  Repeat components 1-3 for the
    duration of the workout.

EFFORT: RPE 5-7
COOL-DOWN: March in place, around your step, and atop your step. Tap the top of your step with alternating feet for 3-5 minutes. Abdominal and back strengthening exercises for 3-5 minutes (optional), then stretch.
APPROXIMATE CALORIES BURNED: 480-560

COMMENTS

To execute heel raises atop the step, stand on the step with feet together. With straight but not locked legs, raise up onto your toes so your heels are elevated. Hold for 2 counts, then lower. For variation, try the same exercise with your knees slightly bent throughout to emphasize the muscles deep within the calf area.

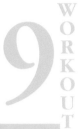

W O R K O U T

TOTAL TIME: 55-65 minutes

WARM-UP: Step on the platform, march on the floor, and alternate toe taps atop the platform while swinging your arms freely using the fullest range of motion for 5 minutes.
BEATS PER MINUTE: 120-126
TIME: 45-50 minutes

MOVEMENTS

Alternate the floor movements with the step movements at your own discretion. Do each component separately, or put them together.

Component 1
Starting position: Side
 March in place with arm reaches.
 *Single lead tap up with pull backs
 *Single lead knee up with fun-time arms
 Over the top 4 times
 March around the step to the other side.
 Repeat * movements.
 Repeat the entire component or proceed to component 2.

Component 2
Starting position: Front
 Alternating basic step with curl ups

Alternating V step with press downs
Alternating power leap up with arm reaches
Step touch on the floor or jumping jack
Repeat, or go on to component 3.

Component 3
Starting position: Side
 Turn step with fun-time arms
 Over the top
 Step touch on the floor
 March all the way around your step.
 Repeat, or go back to component 1.

EFFORT: RPE 5-7
COOL-DOWN: March in place, around your step, and atop your step. Tap the top of your step with alternating feet for 3-5 minutes. Strengthening and stretching exercises for 3-5 minutes.
APPROXIMATE CALORIES BURNED: 360-480

COMMENTS

This is a fun workout. Since you're already familiar with the moves used in this workout, you can really let loose, add your own style, and have a great time!

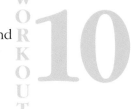

TOTAL TIME: 60-75 minutes

WARM-UP: Step on the platform, march on the floor, and alternate toe taps atop the platform while swinging your arms freely using the fullest range of motion for 5 minutes.
BEATS PER MINUTE: 120-126
TIME: 55-60 minutes

MOVEMENTS

Component 1
Starting position: Side
  March in place with arm reaches.
  *Single lead tap up with pull backs
  *Single lead knee up with fun-time arms
  Over the top 4 times
  March around the step to the other side.
  Repeat * movements.
  Repeat the entire component or proceed to component 2.

Component 2
Starting position: Front
  Alternating basic step with curl ups
  Alternating V step with press downs

  Alternating power leap up with arm reaches
  Step touch on the floor
  Repeat, or go on to component 3.

Component 3
Starting position: Side
  Turn step with fun-time arms
  Over the top
  Step touch on the floor
  March all the way around your step.
  Repeat, or go to component 4.

Component 4
Starting position: Top
  Alternating basic step down
  Alternating lunge
  Alternating tap down
  Repeat, or go back to component 1.

EFFORT: RPE 5-7
COOL-DOWN: March in place, around your step, and atop your step. Tap the top of your step with alternating feet for 3-5 minutes. Strengthening and stretching exercises for 3-5 minutes.
APPROXIMATE CALORIES BURNED: 440-520

COMMENTS

If you enjoy stepping more than you enjoy working out on the floor, adjust the amount of time you spend stepping. For example, do 8 cycles of all step moves in component 2 and only 2 or 4 cycles of step touches on the floor.

Yellow Zone Summary			
Workout	Description	Total duration (minutes)	Intensity (RPE)
1	Combo step interval	50-60	5-7
2	Combo step interval	55-65	5-7
3	Combo step interval	60-75	5-7
4	Long steady step	65-80	5-7
5	Long steady step	70-80	5-7
6	Long steady step	70-80	5-7
7	Toning circuit step	60-70	5-7
8	Toning circuit step	65-80	5-7
9	Combo step fun	55-65	5-7
10	Combo step fun	60-75	5-7

10

Orange Zone

Orange workouts enter the zone of the ultra-exerciser. These workouts are hard.

In this zone, you'll find your perceived exertion ratings hovering in the 8 to 10 range. The duration of these workouts is short, giving you maximum calorie expenditure in the shortest amount of time. The calculations for calorie expenditures are figured based on an individual using a 10-inch step. Using a lower step may result in fewer calories burned. Do not use a higher step because the risk of injury increases. Many of you may find a 10-inch step uncomfortable. Feel free to lower your step height, and increase your intensity through your movement executions instead. Current research recommends 8-inch step heights for most exercisers, with the 10-inch step reserved for athletes and serious exercisers.

Many of the Orange sessions use interval training and incorporate similar workouts as those in chapter 8. The difference in the Orange workouts is clearly the intensity level. To achieve this elevated intensity, we've included some power variations of the movements you're already familiar with. A power version of a traditional step move requires you to add an upward explosive lift, referred to as *propulsion*.

The 10 workouts in this chapter are reserved for the serious, fervent step exerciser who is aiming to reach new heights in fitness by overcoming difficult aerobic, anaerobic, and strength challenges.

Avoid the workouts in this chapter if you experience any discomfort or pain.

COMBO LOW CIRCUIT

WORKOUT 1

TOTAL TIME: 30-40 minutes

WARM-UP: Step on the platform, march on the floor, and alternate toe taps atop the platform while freely swinging your arms using a full range of motion for 5 minutes.

BEATS PER MINUTE: 125-128

TIME: 20-25 minutes

MOVEMENTS

Three minutes of the following power moves:

Starting position: Front

Power V step right lead (1 minute) with curl ups (Leap up with right lead to the corner of the step.)

Power V step left lead (1 minute) with curl ups (Leap up with left lead to the opposite corner of the step.)

Alternating lead basic step (1 minute) with arm reaches

Three minutes of the following power low impact moves:

Alternating power side squats with pull downs

Knee up with arm reaches

Alternating rear lunge with pull downs

Repeat the 3-minute step/3-minute low impact sequences for the duration of the workout.

EFFORT: RPE 8-10

COOL-DOWN: March in place, around your step, and atop your step. Tap the top of your step with alternating feet for 3-5 minutes. Strengthening and stretching exercises for 3-5 minutes.

APPROXIMATE CALORIES BURNED: 180-225

COMMENTS

A new power low impact move is introduced here. To execute the alternating power side squat, start with feet together. With the right foot, step to the right, bending the knees no more than 90 degrees. Hold for 1 count, then leap upward as you return to the starting position. Repeat to the left side. Remember to always concentrate on your posture, form, and execution. Your knees should be aligned over the top of the foot, and your hips and buttocks should extend back and downward as if you were sitting in a chair. Feet remain pointing forward.

COMBO LOW CIRCUIT

TOTAL TIME: 35-45 minutes

WARM-UP: Step on the platform, march on the floor, and alternate toe taps atop the platform while freely swinging your arms using a full range of motion for 5 minutes.
BEATS PER MINUTE: 125-128
TIME: 25-30 minutes

MOVEMENTS

Three minutes of the following power moves:

Starting position: Front
  Power V step right lead (1 minute) with curl ups
  Power V step left lead (1 minute) with curl ups
  Alternating lead basic power step (1 minute) with arm reaches

Three minutes of the following power low impact moves:
  Alternating power side squat with pull downs
  Knee up with arm reaches
  Alternating rear lunge with pull downs

Three minutes of the following power move:

Starting position: Side
  Power leap up with arm reaches (4 repetitions per side)

Repeat the 3-minute step/3-minute low impact step sequences for the duration of the workout.

EFFORT: RPE 8-10
COOL-DOWN: March in place, around your step, and atop your step. Tap the top of your step with alternating feet for 3-5 minutes. Strengthening and stretching exercises for 3-5 minutes.
APPROXIMATE CALORIES BURNED: 225-315

COMMENTS

If you become fatigued during any segment of this workout, you can decrease the intensity by changing the power moves to regular step moves. With each workout though, you should strive to include fewer regular step moves and work toward completing the program as designed.

COMBO HIGH CIRCUIT

TOTAL TIME: 40-50 minutes

WARM-UP: Step on the platform, march on the floor, and alternate toe taps atop the platform while freely swinging your arms using a full range of motion for 5 minutes.
BEATS PER MINUTE: 125-128
TIME: 30-35 minutes

MOVEMENTS

Three minutes of the following power moves:
Starting position: Front
  Power V step right lead (1 minute) with curl ups
  Power V step left lead (1 minute) with curl ups
  Alternating power knee up (1 minute) with arm reaches

Three minutes of the following high impact moves:
  Jogging in place and around the step with pull backs
  Knee up with arm reaches
  Jumping jack with upright rows

Three minutes of the following step moves:
  Alternating knee up with arm reaches
  Turn step with curl ups
  Over the top with fun-time arms

Repeat the 3-minute power step/3-minute high/3-minute step sequences for the duration of the workout.

EFFORT: RPE 8-10
COOL-DOWN: March in place, around your step, and atop your step. Tap the top of your step with alternating feet for 3-5 minutes. Strengthening and stretching exercises for 3-5 minutes.
APPROXIMATE CALORIES BURNED: 270-360

COMMENTS

If you choose to substitute low impact variations for the high impact moves suggested, remember to increase the intensity by concentrating on large, powerful leg movements. For example, the modification for a run would be a march with high knees and arms pumping vigorously. If you like, you can alternate 3 minutes on your favorite piece of aerobic exercise equipment (stair stepping machine, treadmill, stationary bike, etc.) for 1 of the 3-minute cycles.

STEP AND SCULPT

TOTAL TIME: 30-40 minutes

WARM-UP: Step on the platform, march on the floor, and alternate toe taps atop the platform while freely swinging your arms using a full range of motion for 5 minutes.
BEATS PER MINUTE: 125-128
TIME: 20-25 minutes

MOVEMENTS

Alternate 1 minute of step with 1 minute of the strengthening exercise for this entire movement segment.

Starting position: Side
  Alternating power knee up
  Single leg lunge (1 foot atop the step)
  Power turn step with fun-time arms
  Single leg lunge (other foot atop the step)
  Power over the top (Propel your body upward as you go over the top.)
  Power jacks on the floor
  Repeat the sequence for the duration of the workout.

EFFORT: RPE 8-10
COOL-DOWN: March in place, around your step, and atop your step. Tap the top of your step with alternating feet for 3-5 minutes. Abdominal and back strengthening exercises for 3-5 minutes (optional), then stretch.
APPROXIMATE CALORIES BURNED: 180-225

COMMENTS

Power jacks are actually executed as a slow motion jumping jack. Begin with proper posture, feet together and facing forward. Jump up and open your feet as you land (counts 1 and 2). Bend your knees as you're landing to cushion your body from the impact. Now jump up and return to the starting position (counts 3 and 4).

STEP AND SCULPT

5 W O R K O U T

TOTAL TIME: 35-45 minutes

WARM-UP: Step on the platform, march on the floor, and alternate toe taps atop the platform while freely swinging your arms using a full range of motion for 5 minutes.
BEATS PER MINUTE: 125-128
TIME: 25-30 minutes

MOVEMENTS

Alternate 1 minute of step with 1 minute of the strengthening exercises for this entire movement segment.

Starting position: Front
  Alternating power knee up
  Single leg lunge (1 foot atop the step)
  Power turn step with fun-time arms
  Single leg lunge (other foot atop the step)

Starting position: Side
  Power over the top
  Power jack on the floor

Starting position: Top (facing short end)
  Straddle down, power jump up
  Slow alternating lunge
  Repeat the sequence for the duration of the workout.

EFFORT: RPE 8-10
COOL-DOWN: March in place, around your step, and atop your step. Tap the top of your step with alternating feet for 3-5 minutes. Abdominal and back strengthening exercises for 3-5 minutes (optional), then stretch.
APPROXIMATE CALORIES BURNED: 225-315

COMMENTS

Power moves take this workout into the high intensity training zone. Make sure this workout is comfortable, yet challenging.

STEP AND WEIGHTS

TOTAL TIME: 40-55 minutes

WARM-UP: Step on the platform, march on the floor, and alternate toe taps atop the platform while freely swinging your arms using a full range of motion for 5 minutes.
BEATS PER MINUTE: 125-128
TIME: 35-40 minutes

MOVEMENTS

Alternate 1 minute of step with 1 minute of the strengthening exercises (while holding optional weights) for this entire movement segment.

Starting position: Front
  Alternating power knee up
  Single leg lunge (one foot atop the step)
  Power turn step with fun-time arms
  Single leg lunge (other foot atop the step)

Starting position: Side
  Power over the top
  Power jack on the floor

Starting position: Top (facing short end)
  Straddle down, power jump up
  Slow alternating lunge
  Repeat the sequence for the duration of the workout.

EFFORT: RPE 8-10
COOL-DOWN: March in place, around your step, and atop your step. Tap the top of your step with alternating feet for 3-5 minutes. Abdominal and back strengthening exercises for 3-5 minutes (optional), then stretch.
APPROXIMATE CALORIES BURNED: 315-405

COMMENTS

Adding light hand-held weights to the sculpting segment provides a real challenge. Start with 2-pound weights and work your way up to 10 pounds. You can hold the weights at your sides, at your waist, or rest them on your shoulders. Remember to omit the weights during warm-up and cool-down, or if you experience severe discomfort. During step segments weights can be put down or held at your waist if comfortable.

POWER STEP

7

TOTAL TIME: 30-45 minutes

WARM-UP: Step on the platform, march on the floor, and alternate toe taps atop the platform while freely swinging your arms using a full range of motion for 5 minutes.
BEATS PER MINUTE: 125-128
TIME: 20-30 minutes

MOVEMENTS

Starting position: Front
Power basic step right lead with upright rows
3 power turn steps with fun-time arms
Power basic step left lead with upright rows
3 power turn steps with fun-time arms
Slow-motion power over the top with arm reaches
3 power turn steps with fun-time arms
Repeat the sequence for the duration of the workout.

EFFORT: RPE 8-10
COOL-DOWN: March in place, around your step, and atop your step. Tap the top of your step with alternating feet for 3-5 minutes. Strengthening and stretching exercises for 3-5 minutes.
APPROXIMATE CALORIES BURNED: 180-225

COMMENTS

To execute the slow-motion power over the top, allow 2 counts per movement, placing extra concentrated effort on bending the knees to challenge the leg muscles. For example, step atop the platform in 2 counts, squatting through the movement. Then stand atop the platform for the next 2 counts. Step off with 1 foot to the opposite side ending in a squat position for 2 counts. Finally, remove the trail foot from the platform to begin the movement over the top in the other direction.

POWER STEP

TOTAL TIME: 35-45 minutes

WARM-UP: Step on the platform, march on the floor, and alternate toe taps atop the platform while freely swinging your arms using a full range of motion for 5 minutes.
BEATS PER MINUTE: 125-128
TIME: 25-30 minutes

MOVEMENTS

Starting position: Front
  Power basic step right lead with upright rows
  3 power turn steps with fun-time arms
  Power basic step left lead with upright rows
  3 power turn steps with fun-time arms
  Power over the top with arm reaches
  3 power turn steps with fun-time arms
  Power leap up with both lead legs
  Repeat the sequence for the duration of the workout.

EFFORT: RPE 8-10
COOL-DOWN: March in place, around your step, and atop your step. Tap the top of your step with alternating feet for 3-5 minutes. Strengthening and stretching exercises for 3-5 minutes.
APPROXIMATE CALORIES BURNED: 180-225

COMMENTS

This workout uses the same sequences as workout 7. The difference here is the increase in duration. You should have success with this session because the movements are familiar to you.

115

POWER STEP

WORKOUT 9

TOTAL TIME: 40-55 minutes

WARM-UP: Step on the platform, march on the floor, and alternate toe taps atop the platform while freely swinging your arms using a full range of motion for 5 minutes.
BEATS PER MINUTE: 125-128
TIME: 35-40 minutes

MOVEMENTS

Starting position: Front
  Alternating power knee up with variations and arm reaches
  Alternating power V step with curl ups
  Power jump up with arm reaches
  Power turn step with fun-time arms
  Power over the top with upright rows
  Repeat the sequence for the duration of the workout.

EFFORT: RPE 8-10
COOL-DOWN: March in place, around your step, and atop your step. Tap the top of your step with alternating feet for 3-5 minutes. Strengthening and stretching exercises for 3-5 minutes.
APPROXIMATE CALORIES BURNED: 315-405

COMMENTS

Experiment by adding different power movements to the workout once you're familiar with this session's design. Intersperse power and nonpower moves as you see fit. Make it your own!

POWER STEP

TOTAL TIME: 50-60 minutes

WARM-UP: Step on the platform, march on the floor, and alternate toe taps atop the platform while freely swinging your arms using a full range of motion for 5 minutes.
BEATS PER MINUTE: 125-128
TIME: 40-45 minutes

MOVEMENTS

Starting position: Front
  Alternating power knee up with variations and arm reaches
  Alternating power V step with curl ups
  Power jump up with arm reaches
  Turn steps with fun-time arms
  Power over the top with upright rows

Starting position: Top
  Straddle down, power jump up with pull backs
  Alternating lunge with upright rows
  Straddle down, alternating knee up with variations and fun-time arms
  Repeat for the duration of the workout.

EFFORT: RPE 8-10
COOL-DOWN: March in place, around your step, and atop your step. Tap the top of your step with alternating feet for 3-5 minutes. Strengthening and stretching exercises for 3-5 minutes.
APPROXIMATE CALORIES BURNED: 360-450

COMMENTS

This is the most choreographically challenging power routine you'll encounter. Take your time with it. To easily change from the floor to the top of the step, execute half an over the top move, which will get you smoothly into the top position. Feel free to work up to the challenge of putting all the movements together. Remember to integrate power and nonpower moves as you did in workout 9. This workout challenges your body and your mind.

Orange Zone Summary			
Workout	Description	Total duration (minutes)	Intensity (RPE)
1	Combo low circuit	30-40	8-10
2	Combo low circuit	35-45	8-10
3	Combo high circuit	40-50	8-10
4	Step and sculpt	30-40	8-10
5	Step and sculpt	35-45	8-10
6	Step and weights	40-55	8-10
7	Power step	30-45	8-10
8	Power step	35-45	8-10
9	Power step	40-55	8-10
10	Power step	50-60	8-10

11

Red Zone

Think of the Red zone as the workouts that require your greatest efforts. Your intensity will be high and duration long, but the potential rewards are numerous. These workouts have perceived exertion ratings of 8 to 10, and they all last longer than 30 minutes.

The 10 Red sessions will best train the ultra-exerciser who trains hard and is looking for maximum results. The calorie expenditures are calculated based on a 10-inch step height, just as in the previous zone. The workouts will continue to be diverse so you get the most excitement, variety, and motivation. You have the option to add weights to workouts 4 through 6. Weights should be used only for the sculpting segments, not for the step segment. Start with light weights (1 to 3 pounds) and progress to heavier weights (5 to 10 pounds).

Don't attempt these workouts if you're feeling tired or under the weather. It's best to undertake these workouts on nonconsecutive days to allow your body to recover and gear up for the next challenge. During these sessions, it's especially important to have high-energy music to keep you motivated. Good luck!

COMBO HIGH CIRCUIT

1 W
O
R
K
O
U
T

TOTAL TIME: 40-50 minutes

WARM-UP: Step on the platform, march on the floor, jog in place, and alternate toe taps atop the platform while freely swinging your arms using a full range of motion for 5 minutes.
BEATS PER MINUTE: 125-128
TIME: 30-35 minutes

MOVEMENTS

Three minutes of the following moves:

Starting position: Front
 Alternating basic step with curl ups
 Turn step with overhead reaches
 Over the top with fun-time arms
 Alternating knee up with variations and arm reaches

Three minutes of the following moves:
 Jogging in place and around your step
 Jumping jack *or* jumping rope

Three minutes of the following power step moves:

Starting position: Front
 Power V step right leg lead and pull backs (1 minute)
 Power V step left leg lead and upright rows (1 minute)
 Power turn step

Repeat the 3-minute step/high impact/power step sequences for the duration of the workout.

EFFORT: RPE 8-10
COOL-DOWN: March in place, around your step, and atop your step. Tap the top of your step with alternating feet for 3-5 minutes. Strengthening and stretching exercises for 3-5 minutes.
APPROXIMATE CALORIES BURNED: 270-315

COMMENTS

During the high impact segment, challenge yourself to jump rope. Begin by integrating the rope jumping with the other high impact moves. Progress to jumping for the entire 3-minute circuit. This is a great calorie burner!

COMBO HIGH CIRCUIT

TOTAL TIME: 50-60 minutes

WARM-UP: Step on the platform, march on the floor, jog in place, and alternate toe taps atop the platform while freely swinging your arms using a full range of motion for 5 minutes.
BEATS PER MINUTE: 125-128
TIME: 40-45 minutes

MOVEMENTS

Three minutes of the following step moves:

Starting position: Side
  Over the top with upright rows
  Turn step with reaches
  Alternating knee up with variations and curl ups
  Alternating repeater with fun-time arms

Three minutes of the following moves:
  Jogging in place
  Jumping jack
  High impact alternating knee up *or* jump rope

Three minutes of the following power step moves:

Starting position: Front
  Power leap up with arm reaches
  Alternating power knee up with upright rows
  Power jump up with fun-time arms

Repeat the 3-minute step/high impact/power step sequences for the duration of the workout.

EFFORT: RPE 8-10
COOL-DOWN: March in place, around your step, and atop your step. Tap the top of your step with alternating feet for 3-5 minutes. Strengthening and stretching exercises for 3-5 minutes.
APPROXIMATE CALORIES BURNED: 360-450

COMMENTS

Concentrate on maximizing your effort and intensity for each 3-minute segment. Getting through the workout in 3-minute segments provides higher motivation than focusing on the length of the entire session. Get psyched!

COMBO HIGH CIRCUIT

3
W
O
R
K
O
U
T

TOTAL TIME: 60-75 minutes

WARM-UP: Step on the platform, march on the floor, jog in place, and alternate toe taps atop the platform while freely swinging your arms using a full range of motion for 5 minutes.
BEATS PER MINUTE: 125-128
TIME: 50-60 minutes

MOVEMENTS

Three minutes of the following moves:

Starting position: Top
Basic step down right leg lead and arm pull downs (1 minute)
Basic step down left leg lead and arm pull downs (1 minute)
Alternating lunge with upright rows (1 minute)

Three minutes of the following moves:
Jogging around the platform and in place with curl ups
Knee up with arm reaches
Jumping jack with upright rows *or* jump rope

Three minutes of the following power step moves:

Starting position: Front
Alternating power V step with arm reaches
Power leap up with right leg lead and upright rows
Power leap up with left leg lead and upright rows

Repeat the 3-minute step/high impact/power step sequences for the duration of the workout.

EFFORT: RPE 8-10
COOL-DOWN: March in place, around your step, and atop your step. Tap the top of your step with alternating feet for 3-5 minutes. Strengthening and stretching exercises for 3-5 minutes.
APPROXIMATE CALORIES BURNED: 450-585

COMMENTS

Make sure you've got supportive footwear for the Red zone workouts. Your feet and legs may become fatigued if you wear poor shoes. Take time to stretch all the muscles of the lower body after this challenging workout.

STEP AND WEIGHTS

TOTAL TIME: 40-50 minutes

WARM-UP: Step on the platform, march on the floor, jog in place, and alternate toe taps atop the platform while freely swinging your arms using a full range of motion for 5 minutes.
BEATS PER MINUTE: 125-128
TIME: 30-35 minutes

MOVEMENTS

Alternate 1 minute of step with 1 minute of the strengthening exercises with weights for the duration of the workout.

Starting position: Side
  Alternating power knee up with arm reaches
  Single leg stationary lunge (one foot atop the step), weights held in
    hands at hip level or placed on the shoulders
  Power turn step with fun-time arms
  Single leg stationary lunge (opposite foot atop the step) with curl ups
    and weights with each lunge
  Power over the top with upright rows
  Power side squats with press downs with weights

EFFORT: RPE 8-10
COOL-DOWN: March in place, around your step, and atop your step. Tap the top of your step with alternating feet for 3-5 minutes. Abdominal and back strengthening exercises for 3-5 minutes (optional), then stretch.
APPROXIMATE CALORIES BURNED: 270-315

COMMENTS

Use weights with the strengthening exercises, then put them off to the side and out of your way during the step segments. If this becomes troublesome and you choose to use the weights during the step segment, keep them stationary at your waist. Moving your arms in the recommended manner *with weights* increases your risk of injury to the shoulder, elbow, and back. Begin with light weights (1 to 3 pounds) and progress to heavier weights (5 to 10 pounds) as you become stronger. Remember to omit weights during warm-ups and cool-downs.

STEP AND WEIGHTS

5 WORKOUT

TOTAL TIME: 50-60 minutes

WARM-UP: Step on the platform, march on the floor, jog in place, and alternate toe taps atop the platform while freely swinging your arms using a full range of motion for 5 minutes.
BEATS PER MINUTE: 125-128
TIME: 40-45 minutes

MOVEMENTS

Alternate 1 minute of step with 1 minute of the strengthening exercises with weights for this entire movement segment.

Starting position: Top
  Basic step down with power jump up right leg lead and fun-time arms
  Alternating slow lunge with press downs and weights
  Basic step down with power jump up left leg lead and fun-time arms
  Alternating slow lunge with curl ups and weights
  Alternating lunge to the beat of the music using no weights
  Heel raise with upright rows and weights
  Tap down with right leg lead and pull backs
  Alternating power squats with pull downs and weights
  Tap down with left leg lead and upright rows

EFFORT: RPE 8-10
COOL-DOWN: March in place, around your step, and atop your step. Tap the top of your step with alternating feet for 3-5 minutes. Abdominal and back strengthening exercises for 3-5 minutes (optional), then stretch.
APPROXIMATE CALORIES BURNED: 360-450

COMMENTS

To complete the heel raise exercise, stand atop your step with feet together. Raise both heels simultaneously, while keeping your legs and knees straight, but not locked. Hold for 1 count and lower. This is a great calf-shaping exercise.

STEP AND WEIGHTS

W O R K O U T

6

TOTAL TIME: 60-75 minutes

WARM-UP: Step on the platform, march on the floor, jog in place, and alternate toe taps atop the platform while freely swinging your arms using a full range of motion for 5 minutes.
BEATS PER MINUTE: 125-128
TIME: 50-60 minutes

MOVEMENTS

Alternate 1 minute of step with 1 minute of the strengthening exercises for this entire movement segment.

Starting position: Corner
  Alternating power knee up with variations and arm reaches
  Single leg stationary lunge (one foot atop the step) and upright rows
    with weights
  Power turn step with fun-time arms
  Single leg stationary lunge (opposite foot atop the step) and curl ups
    with weights
  Power over the top with pull backs
  Power squat with pull downs and weights

Starting position: Top (facing short end)
  Straddle down, power jump up
  Slow alternating lunge with press downs and weights
  Repeat for the duration of the workout.

EFFORT: RPE 8-10
COOL-DOWN: March in place, around your step, and atop your step. Tap the top of your step with alternating feet for 3-5 minutes. Abdominal and back strengthening exercises for 3-5 minutes (optional), then stretch.
APPROXIMATE CALORIES BURNED: 450-585

COMMENTS

This is a great total-body challenge. Getting stronger through the use of hand weights is a great way to increase your body's calorie burning abilities as well as to shape up your muscles.

POWER STEP

7 WORKOUT

TOTAL TIME: 40-50 minutes

WARM-UP: Step on the platform, march on the floor, jog in place, and alternate toe taps atop the platform while freely swinging your arms using a full range of motion for 5 minutes.
BEATS PER MINUTE: 125-128
TIME: 30-35 minutes

MOVEMENTS

Starting position: Front
Power basic step right leg lead with upright rows
3 power turn steps with fun-time arms
Power basic step left leg lead with upright rows
3 power turn steps with fun-time arms
Slow-motion power over the top
3 power turn steps with fun-time arms
Power jump up
Repeat the sequence for the duration of the workout.

EFFORT: RPE 8-10
COOL-DOWN: March in place, around your step, and atop your step. Tap the top of your step with alternating feet for 3-5 minutes. Strengthening and stretching exercises for 3-5 minutes.
APPROXIMATE CALORIES BURNED: 270-360

COMMENTS

Do you recall the slow-motion power over the top from the Orange zone workout? Here it is again. Remember to concentrate on bending the knees no deeper than 90 degrees throughout the entire sequence. If you need a refresher, review workout 7 from the Orange zone. Alternate nonpower moves as needed.

POWER STEP

TOTAL TIME: 50-60 minutes

WARM-UP: Step on the platform, march on the floor, jog in place, and alternate toe taps atop the platform while freely swinging your arms using a full range of motion for 5 minutes.
BEATS PER MINUTE: 125-128
TIME: 40-45 minutes

MOVEMENTS

Starting position: Front
  Alternating power knee up with variations and arm reaches
  Alternating power V step with curl ups
  Power jump up with arm reaches
  Power turn step with fun-time arms
  Slow-motion power over the top with upright rows
  Repeat for the duration of the workout.

EFFORT: RPE 8-10
COOL-DOWN: March in place, around your step, and atop your step. Tap the top of your step with alternating feet for 3-5 minutes. Strengthening and stretching exercises for 3-5 minutes.
APPROXIMATE CALORIES BURNED: 360-450

COMMENTS

Experiment by adding different power and nonpower movements to the workout, just as you did in the Orange zone. This helps to add variety and empowers you to do your best. Make sure your music motivates you.

MEGASTEP

TOTAL TIME: 40-50 minutes

WARM-UP: Step on the platform, march on the floor, jog in place, and alternate toe taps atop the platform while freely swinging your arms using a full range of motion for 5 minutes.
BEATS PER MINUTE: 125-128
TIME: 30-35 minutes

MOVEMENTS

Divide your workout time into 4 segments. For example, if you're planning a 40-minute workout, each part would be executed for 10 minutes.

Part 1   Step
Starting position: Top (facing short end)
  Alternating straddle down with press downs
  Alternating lunge with arm reaches
  Alternating straddle down, power jump up with press downs
  Alternating lunge with arm reaches
  Repeater lunge (4 per side) with fun-time arms
  Repeat until time has elapsed for part 1.

Part 2   Strengthening with weights
Starting position: Front
  Alternating single leg lunge and curl ups with weights
  Right leg stationary lunge and upright rows with weights
  Left leg stationary lunge and pull downs with weights
  Power side squats with press downs
  Do sets of these exercises until the allotted time has expired. Begin with 8 repetitions per exercise and progress to 15-20 repetitions.

Part 3   High impact
  Jogging in place and around the platform
  Jumping jack
  Alternating knee up
  8 single leg kicks per leg *or* jump rope
  Repeat the movements until the allotted time has expired.

Part 4   Power step
Starting position: Front
  Power V step with right leg lead and curl ups
  Power V step with left leg lead and arm reaches
  Power leap up with right leg lead and upright rows
  Power leap up with left leg lead and upright rows
  Alternating basic step and fun-time arms
  Turn step with pull downs
  Repeat for the duration of this segment.

EFFORT: RPE 8-10
COOL-DOWN: March in place, around your step, and atop your step. Tap the top of your step with alternating feet for 3-5 minutes, then stretch. Abdominals and back strengthening exercises for 3-5 minutes (optional), then stretch.
APPROXIMATE CALORIES BURNED: 270-360

MEGASTEP

TOTAL TIME: 50-60 minutes

WARM-UP: Step on the platform, march on the floor, jog in place, and alternate toe taps atop the platform while freely swinging your arms using a full range of motion for 5 minutes.
BEATS PER MINUTE: 125-128
TIME: 40-45 minutes

MOVEMENTS

Part 1   Step
Starting position: Top (facing short end)
- Alternating straddle down with press downs
- Alternating lunge with arm reaches
- Alternating straddle down, power jump up with press downs
- Alternating lunge with arm reaches
- Repeater lunge (4 per side) with fun-time arms
- Repeat until time has elapsed for part 1.

Part 2   Strengthening with weights
Starting position: Front
- Alternating leg lunge and curl ups with weights
- Right leg stationary lunge and upright rows with weights
- Left leg stationary lunge and pull downs with weights
- Power side squats with press downs
- Do sets of these exercises until the allotted time has expired. Begin with 8 repetitions per exercise and progress to 15-20 repetitions of each exercise.

Part 3   High impact
- Jog in place and around the platform
- Jumping jack
- Alternating knee up
- 8 single leg kicks per leg *or* jump rope
- Repeat the movements until the allotted time has expired.

Part 4   Power step
Starting position: Front
- Power V step with right leg lead and curl ups
- Power V step with left leg lead and arm reaches
- Power leap up with right leg lead and upright rows
- Power leap up with left leg lead and upright rows
- Alternating basic step and fun-time arms
- Turn step with pull downs
- Repeat for the duration of this segment.

EFFORT: RPE 8-10
COOL-DOWN: March in place, around your step, and atop your step. Tap the top of your step with alternating feet for 3-5 minutes. Abdominal and back strengthening exercises for 3-5 minutes (optional), then stretch.
APPROXIMATE CALORIES BURNED: 360-450

Red Zone Summary			
Workout	Description	Total duration (minutes)	Intensity (RPE)
1	Combo high circuit	40-50	8-10
2	Combo high circuit	50-60	8-10
3	Combo high circuit	60-75	8-10
4	Step and weights	40-50	8-10
5	Step and weights	50-60	8-10
6	Step and weights	60-75	8-10
7	Power step	40-50	8-10
8	Power step	50-60	8-10
9	Megastep	40-50	8-10
10	Megastep	50-60	8-10

PART III

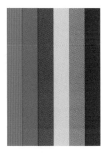

TRAINING BY THE WORKOUT ZONES

Now for the fun part. By now you should be comfortable with the material presented in parts I and II. We now help you put it into a personalized workout program specifically designed to meet your goals.

The programs in part III are based on your abilities and your goals. Use the charts that follow to identify and design your personal program. Your personal program will be based on two foundational premises: your performance level and your long-term goal.

Easy Stepping

If your goal is to get started on a step training program that will enhance your overall well-being, yet won't be too challenging, the Beginning Stepping Program is for you. You'll see slight cardiovascular and body composition changes, as well as some muscular change. You'll probably average three workouts per week.

Moderate Stepping

A moderate step exerciser trains a little more often with a little more intensity. You qualify for the Frequent Stepping Program if you workout four to five times per week and want to burn more calories and see marked improvements in the cardiovascular and musculoskeletal systems. This program will improve your aerobic endurance and body composition if combined with a healthy, low-fat diet.

Challenging Stepping

Here, the emphasis transfers to setting and resetting personal goals for serious training. You'll require more frequent training sessions, higher intensities, and much more commitment. The Ultra-Exerciser Stepping Program, which is appropriate for amateur and professional athletes, will bring significant increases in cardiovascular endurance, muscle power, and calorie expenditure.

Remember, you're never locked into a particular performance category. Feel free to move among the categories as your fitness levels improve and your goals change. Above all, your lifelong good health and well-being and your feelings of accomplishment demand that you choose a training schedule and program that matches your present abilities and ambitions.

12

Setting Up Your Personal Program

When you engage in a safe and challenging training program, your fitness improves. Going a bit beyond what your body is used to doing is termed *overload*. Overload, when used appropriately, can help you meet your fitness goals. For example, if you've been stepping for 25 minutes for the past two months and you feel you've stopped seeing physical changes, pushing to 35-minute step sessions may be enough overload to resume those changes. However, when used inappropriately, overload can actually harm you. Let's suppose you possess enough aerobic endurance to complete a nonstop, steady-state step workout for 30 minutes. You've set a goal to sustain a 60-minute power step workout. Instead of increasing in small increments, you decide to just go for it, and you attempt the power step workout for 60 minutes. Doubling the duration and going from steady-state stepping to power stepping all at once may be too much. As a result of this excessive overload, you're now at a greater risk for injury, excessive fatigue, and a major, but temporary, setback in your program.

Getting what you want out of any training program requires you to systematically apply external stresses so your body can revise its level of fitness with each workout. For example, if you wanted to get stronger biceps (you want the ability to curl 50 pounds, let's say) and your current program had you doing biceps curls with 10-pound weights, you'd need to systematically add increments of 5 pounds to your workout until you finally achieved your goal of curling 50 pounds. Once accomplished, we say your strength level has been revised from being able to curl 10 pounds to being able to curl 50. Each 5 pound increase actually had a building block effect, bringing you to new levels of fitness until you've achieved your ultimate goal.

We outline recommendations in this chapter to provide you with a framework for your training program. These guidelines for fitness testing, tailoring your program, and cross training are applicable for all step exercisers—old or young, male or female, beginner or experienced.

Tune In to Your Body's Messages

Your body is a unique machine that communicates to you when you listen. Did you ever wake up and feel weak and achy, yet you pushed yourself through a workout and ended up with a virus a few days later? Listening to your body and taking that day off might have reduced your risk of suffering from that virus. Problems arise when people aren't tuned in to their bodies or don't know what to do when they sense something is wrong. The best way to prevent unnecessary injury or illness and obtain maximum benefits is to listen to your body and respond to its signals.

You can recognize some of the most critical and apparent signals easily. Your heart rate, body weight, energy level, and hours of sleep help you to clearly interpret your body's messages. For example, an unusually high morning heart rate, low energy levels, or excessive fatigue following training can indicate that your body hasn't quite recovered from your last workout. A significant and quick reduction in body weight can indicate possible dehydration. If you don't get the sleep you need, it will be hard to complete your workouts, no matter what your level is.

To determine if you're pushing beyond your body's capabilities, simply answer these questions each morning:

1. Is your resting pulse, taken before you get out of bed in the morning, 10 percent higher than normal?
2. Is your energy level when you wake up less than normal?
3. Are you waking up exhausted or more fatigued than normal?
4. Did you sleep 10 percent fewer hours last night than normal?

If no is your answer to all these questions, continue with the challenges you've set for yourself. However, if you've answered yes to one question, ease up a bit on your day's workout. If you've answered yes to two or three questions, plan to work out at an easy pace for a short time. Answering yes to all four questions is a good indication that your body needs some time off. When in doubt, be conservative and take a break!

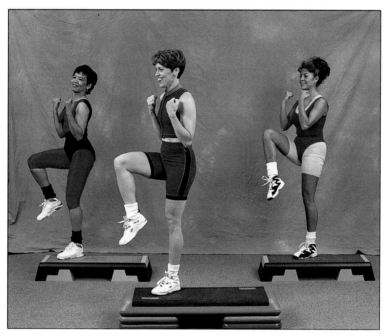

Tuning into your body's messages and tracking your progress will help you achieve your fitness goals.

Setting Personal Goals

How long and how intensely you step is determined by how fit you are. Many methods are available to test various components of fitness, but we recommend the following ones:

Tracking Fitness Progress

The first fitness component that you tested in chapter 3 was your aerobic fitness. Take the test every six months to reevaluate your cardiovascular fitness. As you get in better shape, you will begin to see an improvement in your fitness category.

Another fitness component you can keep track of is your body composition. Body composition is the percentage of lean body mass (muscle) compared to body fat. This can be accurately assessed by an exercise specialist with special equipment and the use of mathematical formulas. However, we have a few simple ways for you to get a rough estimate of your body's changes as you progress.

1. **Waist to hip ratio.** Divide your waist measurement by your hip measurement to get another measure of weight status. A waist to hip ratio greater than 1.0 is an indication that you may be overweight or overfat.
2. **Pinch test.** Remember the pinch test? If you can pinch more than an inch . . . . There may be some validity to this test, although it's crude. This test is based on the same theory as skinfold tests. The pinch test gives you a very rough estimate, however most people can realistically shoot for a goal of pinching two inches or less on their abdomen.
3. **Belt test.** A good sign that you're losing body weight and fat is when you find yourself having to tighten your belt.

Two other important components of health and fitness that you can keep track of are muscular strength and endurance. Muscular *strength* is defined as the greatest amount of force a muscle or group of muscles can produce during one maximal contraction; muscular *endurance* is the ability of a muscle or muscle group to perform repeated contractions for an extended period of time. Muscular strength is the more difficult to assess unless you have a spotter and appropriate weight equipment; however, testing your muscular endurance can be done easily without special equipment. Here are two simple tests for muscular endurance: the push-up test and the curl-up test.

Push-Up Test.   This is a good endurance test for the upper body. To complete the push-up test, follow these four steps:

1. Lie on your abdomen on a padded floor. If you are male, your body should be straight, and your hands should be directly under your shoulders. For females, use the modified push-up test. Lift your feet off the ground while keeping your knees on the floor.
2. Exhale while raising up until your arms are straight. It is important to keep the upper body and torso straight throughout the movement.
3. Lower your chest to within three inches of the floor, and raise back up.
4. Count the total number of nonstop push-ups performed and compare with the norms in the accompanying table.

Table 12.1
Norms for Push-Up Test

Men

Rating	20-29	30-39	40-49	50-59	60+
Excellent	>55	>45	>40	>35	>30
Good	45-54	35-44	30-39	25-34	20-29
Average	35-44	25-34	20-29	15-24	10-19
Fair	20-34	15-24	12-19	8-14	5-9
Poor	<19	<14	<11	<7	<4

Women

Rating	20-29	30-39	40-49	50-59	60+
Excellent	>49	>40	>35	>30	>20
Good	34-48	25-39	20-34	15-29	5-19
Average	17-33	12-24	8-19	6-14	3-4
Fair	6-16	4-11	3-7	2-5	1-2
Poor	<5	<3	<2	<1	0

Curl-Up Test.   The curl-up test also has four parts:

1. Lie on your back on a padded floor mat. Bend your knees and place your feet flat on the floor, 12 to 18 inches from your buttocks.
2. Place your hands on either side of your ears to cradle your head or place your hands across your chest, whichever is more comfortable. Don't push your chin to your chest.
3. Contract your abdominal muscles as you curl your shoulders and upper back upward and forward.
4. Record the number of curl ups completed in 60 seconds and compare to the accompanying table.

Table 12.2 Norms for Bent-Knee Curl-Up Test				
Men				
Rating	**20-29**	**30-39**	**40-49**	**50-59**	**60+**
Excellent	>48	>40	>35	>30	>25
Good	43-47	35-39	30-34	25-29	20-24
Average	37-42	29-34	24-29	19-24	14-19
Fair	33-36	25-28	20-23	15-18	10-13
Poor	<32	<24	<19	<14	<9
Women				
Rating	**20-29**	**30-39**	**40-49**	**50-59**	**60+**
Excellent	>44	>36	>31	>26	>21
Good	39-43	31-35	26-30	21-25	16-20
Average	33-38	25-30	19-25	15-20	10-15
Fair	29-32	21-24	16-18	11-14	6-9
Poor	<28	<20	<15	<10	<5

Flexibility, the last component of fitness, is defined as the range of motion around a joint. A traditional test of flexibility is the sit and reach test. However, this test requires the use of special equipment, so we recommend you use this simpler method that requires only a 12-inch ruler.

Modified Sit and Reach Test.

This test has three parts:

1. Sit with your back and buttocks firmly against a wall with your legs and feet extended straight in front of you, toes pointing toward the ceiling; so your ankle forms a 90-degree angle.
2. Set the zero end of the ruler next to your heel. Lay the ruler on the floor so it acts as an extension of your leg.
3. Without bending your knees or moving the ruler, bend forward at your waist and see how far you can reach. The more flexible you are, the farther down the ruler your reach will extend.

Choose Your Workout Schedule

A variety of workout schedules are provided for you in chapter 13. You can follow our recommendations or design your own program. No matter what you choose to do, take the following steps when tailoring the program to your needs:

1. **Select your goal for your program.** The workouts in this book can help you gain aerobic (cardiovascular) and anaerobic fitness, strengthen your muscles, and help you lose body fat and weight if combined with low-fat, moderate-calorie meal selections. An example of a goal might be a 10 percent decrease in your resting heart rate (a measure of improved cardiovascular fitness).
2. **Select the time available.** By realistically determining how much time you have to devote to your training program, you can determine which workouts will fit into your schedule. For example, you can devote 30 minutes twice a week and 60 minutes twice a week toward achieving your goal.
3. **Select an appropriate starting level.** Depending on your current fitness level, choose a starting point that will be comfortable and not too challenging.
4. **Select an approximate goal date.** Pick a date that's realistic based on consistent progress at a normal pace. Your goal date can be from a few weeks to a few months away. After you get started, you'll know what normal is for your body. Be patient. For example, "I want to have a 10 percent decrease in my resting heart rate in two months."

The programs presented in chapter 13 reflect the two-week rotational cycle. Every two weeks, the cycle changes. First you'll complete three workouts per week, then four, five, and eventually six. This will allow you to get proficient at the workouts while providing training options and variety.

If you choose to deviate from our prescription and design your own plan, we suggest that you still follow these guidelines:

1. Your performance level should determine how much, how often, and how hard you step. If you are a beginner, your workouts will be every other day for an average of 20 to 30 minutes and only one challenging workout per week. The ultra-exerciser, on the other hand, will enjoy training sessions for six days with one or two challenging workouts per week.
2. Your ability, ambition, and level of motivation should determine how challenging your workouts should be. If you're a beginner just starting your training and have never been fond of exercising, keep your workouts short and easy until you're motivated for a challenge.

On the other hand, if you're an avid exerciser with advanced skills, go for the challenge.

3. Take a day or two off after harder workouts (an RPE of 5 or more). If you pushed yourself and stepped longer and more intensely than normal (an RPE of 4 or more), schedule a day or two of active rest (walking, stretching) immediately following. Don't ever work out hard two days in a row. Recovery is the key to successful workouts.

Starting Level

Knowing how hard and how much exercise to do when first starting out is the hardest fitness training decision to make. The simplest philosophy to follow is to start out at a low intensity and duration and progress gradually. If you have not been very active in the past, start out with the Green or Blue workouts. Gradually progress to the other workout zones as you feel your strength and endurance improving. Remember, the first reason people drop out of an exercise program is because they do too much too fast, and they eventually get extremely frustrated, fatigued, or injured. You may need to start out with a simple 10- to 15-minute workout at a low intensity. Feel free to adjust the workouts to meet your needs. Use our color-coded system as your road map. Road maps, like our workouts, have a variety of alternate routes, all eventually leading to your destination. We're flexible, and you should be too.

Cross-Training Options

Step training is one of a number of workout methods that help you achieve fitness. We suggest that you mix and match fitness activities. This is where cross training comes in. The following list gives some important reasons to include cross training in your program:

1. It provides a substitute activity during injury periods. By overspecializing, you run the risk of physical injury. When you've suffered an injury from overuse or some other means, it's important to have some type of alternative exercise, such as swimming or calisthenics, that won't aggravate the problem.
2. It relieves boredom when your step routines temporarily fail to stimulate your interests. Substituting another activity for a few days or weeks can restore your spark to step again.
3. It provides rest-day physical activities. Step training workouts require a break from their up-and-down effects on the body. A leisurely walk or bike ride provides great cross-training benefits and enjoyment on your rest days.

Overall, cross training provides active, recreational rest and recovery. To accomplish this, these supplemental workouts should be recreational, low in intensity, and brief in duration.

Strength Training

As mentioned earlier, stepping can not only result in tight muscles, but it can also develop certain muscles while limiting the strength in others. The lower body becomes relatively strong, whereas the upper body (if not specifically targeted in the workouts) goes virtually unexercised.

Because these strength imbalances can lead to injuries, we recommend that you add the strength exercises presented in chapter 5 to your program. Although we suggest simple exercises in chapter 5 that require minimal equipment, you can engage in a more complex routine incorporating free weights and cardiovascular equipment. Some of the more popular cardiovascular equipment is available at health clubs, gyms, and at retail stores for the home market. You can choose from treadmills, stationary bicycles, stair steppers, health riders, slide boards, ski machines, and much more. In addition some other options are described in the following paragraphs.

Aerobics Classes (Land or Water)

The variety of aerobics classes available today is vast. Choose from low impact, aqua, funk, boxing, martial arts, slide, country line dancing, and many others. Aerobics trains most major muscle groups, but you should beware of high impact exercises that can increase your risk of injury due to their repetitive pounding. Aqua aerobics is an excellent activity because it provides a challenging workout with virtually no risk of injury from weight bearing stress.

Biking (Street or Stationary)

Biking off or on roads gets you outdoors. Enjoying the fresh air and scenery while getting a workout is satisfying and enjoyable. Biking allows you to explore twice as much terrain as you would while walking or running.

Stationary biking lacks the benefits of traveling, but it does provide the same no-impact workout. And on a stationary bike you don't have the threats of traffic, bad weather, or your own carelessness.

Swimming

The advantage of swimming over stepping (besides its being no-impact), is that it exercises more of the body while promoting flexibility.

The disadvantage of swimming is its tendency toward sensory deprivation. It's hard to include music, scenery, and friends. Many refer to pool workouts as being in solitary confinement.

Walking

Walking is the most available and most popular way to train. According to the National Sporting Goods Association's 1992 report, nearly 70 million people participated in walking workouts. You can walk anywhere, anytime, and with very little risk of developing impact-related injuries.

Walking is an efficient exercise, but it tends to be low in intensity. The benefits from walking are slower to come than with other cross-training activities, unless you are race walking. Therefore, you must walk longer to achieve the same benefits.

How Often and How Long Should You Cross Train?

We recommend limiting most of your rest or recovery cross-training sessions to 30 minutes a couple times per week, so you won't drain your energy from your next day's step training. A 30-minute bike ride or aerobics class is about equal in energy expenditure to a 30-minute step workout, provided the intensity levels are about the same. Remember your cross-training workout should be physically, mentally, and emotionally refreshing.

13

Sample Stepping Programs

It's very difficult to prescribe one training regimen for everyone, so we've decided to offer a multitude of choices in this chapter. You'll notice a variety of schedules covering the three levels of performance: beginner, frequent exerciser, and ultra-exerciser.

Each four-week program provides you with a well-balanced, diverse program that leads to improvements in cardiorvascular fitness, anaerobic fitness, and strength fitness.

Beginning Stepping Program

Beginning steppers are often referred to as *novices*. As a novice stepper, you'll probably be interested in obtaining aerobic and body composition changes in addition to an overall feeling of well-being.

The schedule of workouts revolves around a three-day-a-week training program. Usually, only one of the workouts will reach into the Orange zone (high intensity, short duration). The remaining workouts fall into the low intensity Green and Blue zones, and the medium intensity Purple and Yellow zones.

As a novice stepper, you aren't expected to begin these programs unprepared. Spend a week or two acclimating yourself to the step and its basic movements and exercises. Attempt to work your way up to a rehearsal session of approximately 15 to 20 minutes without fatigue before attempting the schedules presented here. Remember the importance of listening to your body.

Easy Does It I

This four-week cycle will give you a structured program that exposes you to a variety of step workouts. Pay careful attention to what types of workouts are most pleasing to you. The schedule here will act as a primer for more vigorous schedules to come.

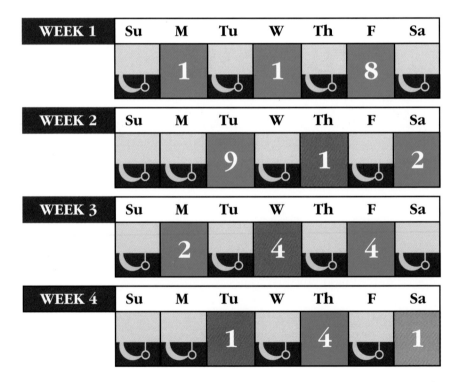

Easy Does It II

This four-week training schedule sets the pace for continued progress. It will prepare you for your transition to the frequent exerciser's training regimen.

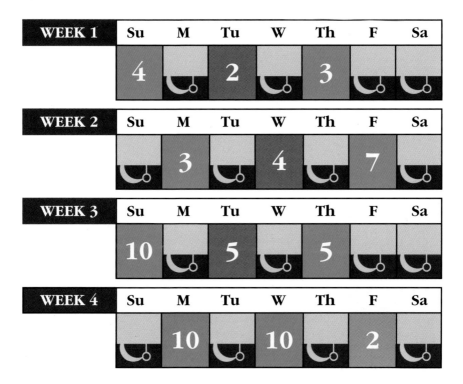

WEEK 1	Su	M	Tu	W	Th	F	Sa
	4		2		3		

WEEK 2	Su	M	Tu	W	Th	F	Sa
		3		4		7	

WEEK 3	Su	M	Tu	W	Th	F	Sa
	10		5		5		

WEEK 4	Su	M	Tu	W	Th	F	Sa
		10		10		2	

Frequent Stepping Program

Frequent stepping takes you beyond exercising for general health benefits. These workouts go a bit longer and push you a bit harder than those workouts recommended for beginners. Frequent exercisers usually are highly motivated and are passionate about doing more than the minimum amounts. They enjoy exploring new and exciting ways to challenge their current levels of fitness.

The workout schedules that follow offer, on average, four to five workouts per week, one of the workouts reaches into the high intensity Orange (short duration) or Red (long duration) zone. The remaining sessions are divided among the other four zones of low and medium intensity.

Rev It Up I

This four-week cycle of training lays the foundation for frequent stepping and provides a variety of workouts. The schedule will also prepare you for your progression to the five-day-a-week program that follows.

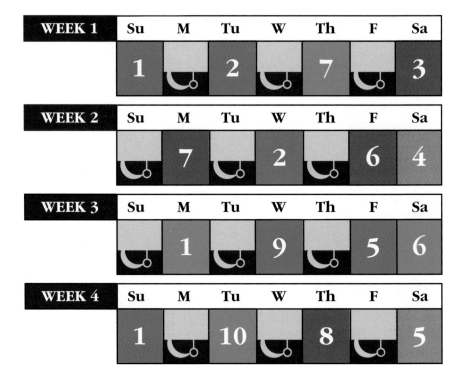

WEEK 1	Su	M	Tu	W	Th	F	Sa
	1		2		7		3

WEEK 2	Su	M	Tu	W	Th	F	Sa
		7		2		6	4

WEEK 3	Su	M	Tu	W	Th	F	Sa
		1		9		5	6

WEEK 4	Su	M	Tu	W	Th	F	Sa
	1		10		8		5

Rev It Up II

This four-week cycle challenges you with workouts that last longer than 50 minutes. The schedule also prepares you for the Rev It Up III program.

WEEK 1	Su	M	Tu	W	Th	F	Sa
	10	3	8		6		2

WEEK 2	Su	M	Tu	W	Th	F	Sa
		4	7		10		1

WEEK 3	Su	M	Tu	W	Th	F	Sa
	9	8		6		1	4

WEEK 4	Su	M	Tu	W	Th	F	Sa
		1	1	7		2	

Rev It Up III

This four-week cycle alternates four- and five-time-a-week workouts, providing you with a lot of versatility and diversity. The schedule prepares you for making the transition to the ultra-exerciser program.

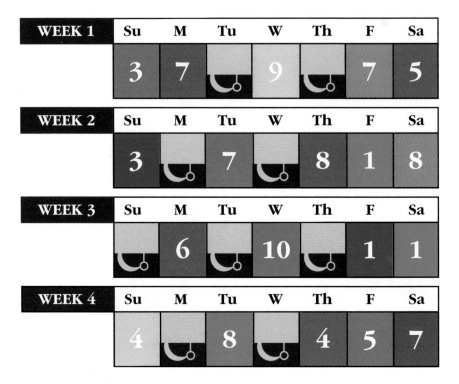

The Ultra-Exerciser Stepping Program

You'll find yourself quite challenged with the training schedules presented here. All schedules suggest training five and six days a week and aim to improve your aerobic fitness, anaerobic fitness, and strength. You'll add weights to the conditioning components, and you'll increase the intensity (RPEs ranging from 7 to 10), and duration (workouts last more than an hour). A few of the workouts in each schedule will reach into the high intensity Orange (short duration) or Red (long duration) zone. The remaining workouts are from the four zones of low to medium intensity. When using the six-day-a-week schedule, pay careful attention to how your body feels, especially your knees and back, to gauge overuse.

Crank It Up

This four-week cycle of training involves working out five days a week. There are two schedules provided for you. Feel free to mix and match them to meet your needs. For example, you could choose the week 1 program from schedule A and the week 2 program from schedule B. These schedules will prepare you for the ultimate six-days-a-week program to follow.

SCHEDULE A

WEEK 1	Su	M	Tu	W	Th	F	Sa
	2	7	2	(rest)	3	(rest)	4

WEEK 2	Su	M	Tu	W	Th	F	Sa
	5	2	(rest)	5	(rest)	10	4

WEEK 3	Su	M	Tu	W	Th	F	Sa
	(rest)	9	4	6	(rest)	6	1

WEEK 4	Su	M	Tu	W	Th	F	Sa
	1	(rest)	6	7	(rest)	6	4

SCHEDULE B

WEEK 1	Su	M	Tu	W	Th	F	Sa
	4	6		8		7	1

WEEK 2	Su	M	Tu	W	Th	F	Sa
	10		3		2	2	4

WEEK 3	Su	M	Tu	W	Th	F	Sa
		3	4	1		10	5

WEEK 4	Su	M	Tu	W	Th	F	Sa
	1		10		6	1	10

The Ultimate Challenge

This cycle of training involves working out six days a week. There are two schedules for you to follow, depending on your needs. Once again, feel free to mix and match the workouts, but be aware of overuse signs such as excessive fatigue or weakness, knee joint pain, or low back pain. We also recommend taking some time for active rest following this 4-week training cycle. For example, a week of walking or biking during week five is a great way to maintain the fitness level you've achieved while giving your body and mind a break from the rigors of the training schedule in this program.

SCHEDULE A

WEEK 1	Su	M	Tu	W	Th	F	Sa
	8	5	8	6	1	1	

WEEK 2	Su	M	Tu	W	Th	F	Sa
	8	4		1	10	10	1

WEEK 3	Su	M	Tu	W	Th	F	Sa
	1		4	1	10	1	4

WEEK 4	Su	M	Tu	W	Th	F	Sa
	1	2		9	3	8	4

SCHEDULE B

WEEK 1	Su	M	Tu	W	Th	F	Sa
	10	1	4		1	6	1

WEEK 2	Su	M	Tu	W	Th	F	Sa
	7	1	4	6	2	4	

WEEK 3	Su	M	Tu	W	Th	F	Sa
	10	1	1	1		10	7

WEEK 4	Su	M	Tu	W	Th	F	Sa
	8	5		2	5	5	3

14

Charting Your Progress

Whether your goal in stepping is for general overall fitness, specific weight management, or improved cardiovascular strength and endurance, keeping track of your progress is easy.

For general overall fitness, you'll know if you're working toward your goal when you assess how your body looks, how your energy level has improved, and even how your daily attitude and sleeping patterns have improved.

If your goal is primarily to manage your weight and body fat, you'll know if step training is helping each time you step on the scale or pull out that tape measure.

Cardiovascular strength and endurance can easily improve and help supply you with more energy and endurance throughout the day. You can measure your progress toward this goal by checking your resting pulse (assessed in the morning when you first awaken). You'll notice how it becomes stronger and slower as your fitness improves. Other fitness tests can be found in chapter 12.

You can even set specific time and intensity goals for yourself. Say your goal is to increase the length of time you spend stepping per week. You'll know if you've accomplished this goal as soon as you add up your weekly workout times. You *will* reach your goals and see changes in your performance and your physique, regardless of your age, gender, and initial level of fitness.

But these changes don't come instantly. They are long-term alterations that occur over time, as the body slowly adapts to the work you're asking it to do. It would be wonderful if we could promise you results overnight, in a week, or in a month. The reality is that changes start to happen, with a regular commitment, after six to eight weeks.

Fitness can't be stored. Stop for as little as a few weeks and the benefits begin to vanish. Keep stepping, or start back up again, and the benefits continue. When you begin to see the changes you desire, or you reach the goals you initially set, it's time to reset, modify, and upgrade. But how do you know? By keeping records, of course. We recommend that you keep a diary, journal, or log of your workouts. That way you're able to measure your progress and compare it against your goal.

You can quickly and easily assess time, weight, body measurements, and pulse. By writing them down today, you can compare them to what you'll soon be achieving. Then you'll know how close you're getting to your goal.

Your personal record keeping system can be as simple as making notes on a calendar or on a sheet of notebook paper or as elaborate as keeping a workout journal or using a commercially available computer program. *How* you keep your records doesn't matter, just make sure to keep them!

Types of Record Keeping

The two types of records you can keep are performance results and physical readings.

Performance Results

At the very least, log the length of time for each workout. Other entries can include the type of workout (steady, circuit, interval) and how you felt (RPE).

Specifically compare the harder workouts that may occur anywhere from once every two weeks for beginning steppers to twice per week for advanced steppers. These are designed with timed intensity intervals to give you a good indication of your performance status and progress.

Completed Performance Log Sample — Rev It Up I Program

	Date	Pulse	Workout color zone	Number	Time (minutes)	RPE	Comments
Su	3/1	72	Blue	1	45	4	Fun workout
M	Day off						
Tu	3/3	70	Blue	2	45	4	Feeling strong today
W	Day off						
Th	3/5	70	Green	7	40	3	Tired
F	Day off						
Sa	3/7	68	Purple	3	55	6	Great energy! Yeah

Weekly summary ___ I felt sluggish and tired during the middle of the week, but regained my energy by the weekend. Overall I had a great week, burned a lot of calories, and feel great.

Physical Readings

Listen to your body. It knows best and tells you how your training is going. Get in the habit of taking 15 seconds to record your resting pulse each morning as you awaken. A decrease in that reading, over time, means that your cardiovascular fitness is improving.

A sudden increase of five beats or more can mean you're getting sick or you're overtrained. Either indicates you need to rest. By logging your heart rate regularly, you'll know what your norm is so you can act appropriately when it appears abnormal.

Also, record your weight and body measurements once a week. Attempt to take these measurements on the same day and at the same time. You may weigh up to five pounds more at night than you do in the morning, so try to avoid being focused on the scale since many things influence fluctuations in weight.

Log Sheets

To get yourself familiar with keeping records, we've included sample log sheets for physical and performance assessment.

Write down the color and number of your planned workout on the performance log sheet. As you complete the workouts, fill in the remaining columns. As in the previous sample, you can use the comments section to record special conditions as well as how you felt.

No matter what you log on your charts or in your journals, your major emphasis should be on continuing your stepping program and feeling good. We want you to profit from the benefit of this fun-filled, successful program for life.

Physical Assessment Log

Week	Day of week/Time	Weight/ A.M. pulse	Girth			Comments/Feelings
			Right thigh/ Left thigh	Bust	Waist	
1						
2						
3						
4						
5						
6						
7						
8						

8-week self-assessment _____

_____

Performance Log

Date	Pulse	Workout color zone	Number	Time (minutes)	RPE	Comments/Feelings
Su						
M						
Tu						
W						
Th						
F						
Sa						

Weekly summary _____

_____

_____

Index

About the Authors

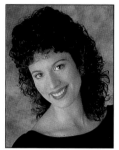

Debi Pillarella, MEd, is the owner of BodyWorks, Inc., and consultant to a number of fitness and health programs. She is also the program developer for FIRST (Fitness Instructor Resource School Training). A fitness professional since 1980, Debi has focused on teaching step aerobics since 1989. She has choreographed and starred in numerous videos on step exercise, including *BodyWorks Step Right Up*, which she also directed and produced, as well as *Step Right Up*, and *Shape* magazine's *Totally Legs* and *Legs, Legs, Legs*.

Debi has received numerous awards in her field. In 1985 she was recognized both as a Certified Fitness Professional by the Aerobics and Fitness Association of America (AFAA) and as a Gold Certified Fitness Professional by the American Council on Exercise. In 1990, she received an award of excellence for the video *Energy Explosion* from the AFAA. In 1993, she was awarded the Certificate of Merit for Fitness Programming by *Fitness Management* magazine. And, in 1996, she was honored for her educational expertise by *Who's Who in American Education*.

Recognized by the International Association of Fitness Professionals (IDEA) as a three-star presenter, Debi travels extensively to train fitness instructors and conduct seminars and workshops on step exercise. Most recently, she coordinated IDEA's new *Becoming a Group Exercise Leader Program*, of which step exercise is a major part.

Debi is the author of several articles on fitness, including her contribution to AFAA's official text, *Fitness Theory and Practice*, a guide to group exercise programs used by more than 20,000 fitness instructors.

Debi is a member of the American College of Sports Medicine and IDEA. In addition, she is on the advisory board of *ACE Certified News*, a publication of the American Council on Exercise. She lives in Chicago, Illinois, with her husband, Jim, and their son, Joseph Nicholas, and enjoys walking, running, strength training, computers, and reading in her spare time.

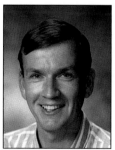

Scott O. Roberts, PhD, a fitness expert and personal trainer, has been involved in the fitness and exercise field since 1986. Scott's work has been recognized by *Fitness Management* magazine and *Who's Who in American Education*.

Scott earned a BS from California State University at Chico, an MS in exercise physiology from CSU at Sacramento, and recently completed his PhD in exercise physiology. He has served as a member of the ACE committees for Personal Training and Aerobic Dance Exercise.

Roberts is the author of several books and articles on fitness training, including *The Business of Personal Training, Strength and Weight Training for Young Athletes*, and *Fitness Walking and Exercise Physiology: Exercise, Performance, and Clinical Applications*. He also has contributed chapters to both the ACE Personal Trainer and Aerobic Dance Instructor manuals, as well as for the AFAA Fitness Instructor Manual.

Scott enjoys exercise, music, and spending time with his wife, Julia, and their three children, Andrew, Daniel, and Michael, in Lubbock, Texas.

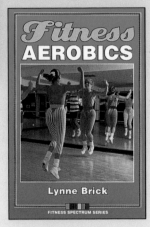
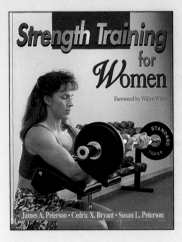